But I Didn't Know
I was Dead!

Walter Willanger

Acacia Publishing

Library of Congress Control Number: 2011963251

ISBN 978-1-935089-52-0

Cover design by Walter Willanger and Jason Crye.
Photos courtesy of Sindre Productions.

Published by Acacia Publishing, Inc.
Gilbert, Arizona
www.acaciapublishing.com

Printed and bound
in the United States of America

Acknowledgments

I would like to express my love and gratitude to the following people. First of all, to my wife, Dolores, and to my family and friends whose love and courage have made my recovery possible; to the paramedics who responded to the emergency immediately and were swift and efficient; to the doctors and medical staff who worked on me, using all their skills in trying to save my life; and to the emergency room nurse who, against all odds, persisted with CPR after I was declared dead because she felt that my soul was still near. Her strong faith restored life in me. For all of these people, I wish to thank them each for the part they played in my miracle.

Chapter 1

It has taken me awhile to write this because I wanted to gather all the information that was available to me so that the story would be correct and accurate. I know it's going to be difficult for me to air so much of my clean as well as dirty laundry, but I will try. My life has been full of events both good and bad so it was difficult to find a starting point but the story you are about to read is true. Many of the names of the people in this story have been omitted due to my respect for other people's privacy. But, if needed for authenticity, they will be disclosed.

First, let me tell you a little bit about myself. My name is Walter and that is my real name. I retired a few years ago, I am past 75 years of age and am of Scandinavian heritage. It was not necessarily my choice, but I was baptized and confirmed as a protestant in the Lutheran religion. As a young boy, I never thought much about anything other than what was going on at the moment. We spent much of our free time playing hide and seek in the summer and sledding on the ice in the winter. Most of our toys were home-made or hand-me-downs from siblings and neighbors. Our schools were occupied from 1940 to 1945 and were made into housing for some of the German troops that were stationed in Norway. My friends and I were very naïve of the world around us; we were just children. I remember one day early in the war. It was winter and there was a lot of snow. My friend and I were walking by our school. Next to the school entrance stood a German soldier on guard, tapping his feet together trying to stay warm. He was in full winter uniform and armed with a rifle and fixed bayonet. As we walked by, I noticed a lot of frost on his bayonet. I then whispered to my friend, "Anyone stuck with a cold bayonet like that would freeze to death." It never entered my mind that freezing would be the least of one's trouble.

Other types of entertainment for us consisted of going through the neighborhood in search of discarded empty milk and soda bottles that we could take back to the store and get a deposit. We didn't get much, but there wasn't much to spend the money on anyway. We would save what we got until we had enough money for a movie ticket. I also remember a time or two when I was asked by my friends to join them at the movie theater, something exciting was playing. As I searched for my money in its hiding place, I was sometimes surprised to find it missing and then find out that my sister was at the movie theater with her friends. This was very disappointing and disturbing to me but in time I got over it, and it forced me to think of better and more clever hiding places.

Another popular thing my friends and I did when we had the opportunity was to go to the library and read books or listen to stories read aloud to us by librarians. One of my fondest memories of that time was one day when I was one of the lucky kids in my school who was picked to spend a few weeks in the summer on a farm far away from the city and the memories of war. I still remember how nice it was to be there and how well they took care of me. They took me on hikes way up in the mountains showing me where they took the cattle to spend the summer months getting fat and how to identify wild animals. They showed me how to make things, including how to fish for trout with homemade fishing gear. But the war was never far away.

One day the farmer asked me if I would like to see an airplane that had been shot down and crashed. Sure, what kid would not want to see that? We hiked and walked it seemed for hours until we came to a big, flat, dry meadow in the mountain. There right in front of us was a large twin-engine airplane pretty much intact. I remember that there was a lot of live ammunition and sharp pieces of aluminum scattered around on the ground. The cockpit was still in one piece and the front section of the airplane was covered with broken glass. I suppose the glass section must have been made of some type of Plexiglas or celluloid for some of it had burned. I was not sure what type of aircraft it was because I did not remember the markings but what I did remember were the wings and cockpit. Years later I figured out that the airplane must have been a German Heinkel 111. The memories from that summer were very special to me and are tucked away forever.

Chapter 2

But as everything else goes, all good things must come to an end and soon I found myself among a lot of kids on the train heading for home. I don't remember much of the train ride other than between every other passenger car there was a flat car and on each flat car there were manned anti-aircraft batteries, I suppose ready to take on any unidentified aircraft in sight.

I must have looked funny waiting for my mother at the train station platform in Oslo with a large name and address label hung over my neck. I had a lot to carry; along with my small suitcase they had also sent a parcel of smoked food for the family. Thankfully my mother found me quickly among all the other kids, otherwise the food may have wound up on someone else's table. On the way home, my mother kept whispering, asking me what was in the two packages that I was carrying. I totally ignored her questions because sitting directly across from us were two German soldiers who were talking and laughing. I was very concerned that everyone on the streetcar could smell the food, and probably wondered where and how I got it.

Besides the food parcel, I had a large paper bag that was ripping apart. Inside was a crudely-made airplane that had British markings scribbled on the wings. My childish fear was that the soldiers would see the airplane with the markings and we would be in trouble. They might send for the police or even the Gestapo. But it all turned out good and I was happy to be back home in a sort of secure environment. The fairytale was now over and it was back to reality and the humdrum existence of war for me and the grownups.

It didn't take long before we learned the habits of war. We knew that when there was a full moon, there would be air raids so that was something we always prepared ourselves for. I spent many nights in air-raid shelters with my mother and sister, waiting for the all-clear sirens to blow. The air attacks were scary in the beginning but we got used to them.

I remember one day in particular. I was at the library when I overheard some of the adults talking about a big apartment house that was hit by bombs during one of the air raids. I didn't hear which city but I did hear that a lot of people had died, though not from the collapse of the apartment building. They had died from drowning. How could that be? I wondered. Then I found out that they had drowned from the broken water pipes that filled up the basement with water. The rubble from the house being bombed had kept them from escaping by blocking their exit. Then I realized that all the pipes, water, sewer and electrical wires in our building also came through the basement where our air-raid shelter was located. So, now I thought the safest place we knew could also be a death trap if our building ever got hit. I told my mother that I would not seek safety in the basement air-raid shelter anymore. From that time on, we took our chances and stayed wherever we were.

For us kids, there was a reward at the end of each air attack. We figured out that all the grenades that were used to shoot at the airplanes had to come down to earth somewhere after they exploded. We would then spend the following days and weeks looking for shrapnel that we could and would use for trading between us kids.

While I'm on the subject of air raids, I would like to include one incident that my friend and I witnessed. It happened during a very quiet holiday, New Year's weekend, I believe. I was playing in the park with one of my very good friends when all of a sudden several airplanes came screaming out of nowhere at a very low altitude above our heads and disappeared into the distance, closely followed by German pursuit fighters. My friend and I probably looked like a couple of question marks after that. What was going on? we thought. Then when the air-raid sirens came on, we started to run for home. While we were running, we noticed that there was a lot of smoke far away in the city. When I got home, there was no one there but I did find a note from my mother that said, "We will be home before dark."

The hours went by and when it started to get dark I got scared. The latest rumor in our neighborhood was that a street car was hit by a bomb. Then we heard that it came from our area and all onboard were killed. What I found out later was that my mother and sister were traveling on that street car but got off two stops before the air raid. They were walking when the bombs hit and then had to take cover in one of the many air-raid shelters in the city and weren't released until late evening.

A couple of weeks later, I had an opportunity to cycle downtown. The route I took allowed me to bike close to the bombed area. I was able to see what was bombed and what damage had been incurred. Years later, I learned that the planes were British twin-engine Mosquitoes. They were on a mission to bomb and destroy the Gestapo headquarters in downtown Oslo. The archives there were supposed to have contained names and addresses of boys 18 years of age and older who would be rounded up by the Gestapo and put into German forced labor camps if needed. But the mission failed. The bombs struck and destroyed an office building, the street car and the rest landed and exploded in the Royal Park next to the palace. The archives were then moved to a safer place only to be destroyed later by Norwegian saboteurs.

Memories of some of the events that happened so long ago are now starting to fade, so it takes a little longer for me to make them resurface. I remember one day in particular close to the end of the war, when our whole neighborhood shook as if there was an earthquake. What had happened was that a ship full of ammunition had blown up. There were fires that raged on throughout the area and there were secondary explosions all over. It was very frightening and I was sure that we would not survive. As a young boy, that was the first time the thought of death ever crossed my mind. Death was something that happened to other people, not to us. I wondered how it felt to die and how I would know I was dead, a question that I suspect many of us have thought of.

Chapter 3

Eventually the war ended and the country started to move toward a full recovery. Things that we hadn't seen on the store shelves in years, such as food, clothing, household merchandise and a few luxury items, slowly became available. There were no more queues for me to stand in. I no longer had to be afraid and embarrassed of being told to leave when I got to the front of the line because we were not regular customers. I later figured out that those few potatoes or whatever other edible things they had were only for sale to the store owners' neighbors and friends. Now that the war was over, I saw several of the same people pointing fingers at anyone else suspected of having had anything to do with the black market or who, in their opinion, had not resisted the occupying forces enough.

The few German soldiers that I saw were all in small groups, disarmed and wearing white arm bands. There were lots of strange and different people everywhere, some wearing uniforms and speaking languages that I had never heard before, others in civilian clothing with identifying markings painted or sewn on. The markings, I was told, were to let people know that they had spent the war years in a concentration camp, prison, or were out of the country on military duty. This was an easy way to identify people and to ask or inquire about other people who had been in work camps and were still missing.

One day, I was told by my mother that my father was coming for a visit. I was very excited to see him since I really didn't know what he was like or what he looked like. The last time I had seen my father was before the war and then I was not even five years old; now I was ten. I was sort of fantasizing, hoping that I would be able to show him off to my friends because for the last five years, my sister and I were the only kids in our neighborhood who didn't have a father around. At times, I would be very embarrassed when the subject of fathers came up. I would tell my friends that someday my father would come, you will see. Little did I know that one of the reasons he was not around was that he had spent years in a German prisoner of war camp.

My father was a marine pilot by occupation and also had the Navy rank of Lieutenant Commander. At the start of the war, when the German military began to expand northward, the British and the French arrived in Norway to help and assist the Norwegians in halting the Germans. The ship my father was assigned to was a French warship. The battle for Narvik took place on April 9, 1940 and it turned out to be one of the first and biggest sea battles at the start of World War II. The Allied Forces were not strong enough to halt the German military. The battle raged on for several days and the ship my father was assigned to was eventually destroyed and sunk. He was picked up by the Germans and was now a prisoner of war. Since he was a Norwegian citizen and a marine pilot and was very familiar with the area, he was directed by the Germans to help them follow and catch the fleeing Allied

Forces. From the information that I read in the newspaper years after the war, he gave the German Commander the wrong coordinates. The ship that he was on then ran aground and was badly damaged and many of those Allied warships that they were following got away. For this he was awarded the medal Croix de Guerre, the highest recognition given by the French government to a non-French citizen.

Chapter 4

As I mentioned earlier, the post-war years were very stressful; there were so many changes and so much chaos to deal with. It was about that time that I found out that my father and mother were divorced or getting a divorce. I didn't know which it was. I was not even 11 years old yet but I did feel that there was some type of custody battle going on between them, which resulted in me going with my father to stay with my grandmother way up north about 200 miles above the Arctic Circle. I arrived at my 82-year old grandmother's home in the middle of winter. She was very kind and good to me and soon got me enrolled in school where I made lots of new friends. I still missed my mother and sister very much and wrote letters to them weekly, but as time went on it got better.

I remember getting a flashlight so I could find my way around the village. At that time of the year, there was twilight for only a couple hours a day then it became dark again. But the evenings and nights were something else. The Northern Lights (Aurora Borealis) were flashing across the sky several times a week. To us kids that was very exciting because we had been told by some of the older kids that if you wave a white handkerchief at the light, it will get mad and come down and get you. To check out the story, we found a good, safe hiding place and then we took turns walking away from it, pretending we didn't see the Northern Lights. Then suddenly we would wave a white handkerchief at it and run as fast as we could to safety. I think among all the fun things we did as children, this was the most fun as well as the scariest.

We did a lot of other things too; some were very stupid but always exciting. At times when there was ice in the bay, we would find an ice floe that was big enough to stay afloat with a kid standing on it. It was quite a challenge because if we got too far to the edges, the ice floe would tip over and dump us into the freezing sea water. The fun part was to navigate around close to shore with a long pole touching the bottom and pretending that we were grown up sailors. There were also war-time bunkers and equipment around the area that we had access to and would become our play area. I remember a ship that had been torpedoed nearby. It sank quickly, close to shore in the shallow water. Two of the masts and the stack were always visible above the water but the bridge could only be seen at low tide. I was told that the ship went to the bottom so fast that some of the crew who were below deck drowned while trying to escape through the small portholes. Although the ship was immediately stripped of anything of value, it was now just another war-time navigational hazard. I was always uncomfortable being near that ship. After about a year, I think the responsibility of having to care for me became too much for my father and grandmother. Custody was again changed. I was returned to my mother and I again left my friends up north for a new life in Oslo. My sister and I only had a few visits from our father after I returned back home. My father never got to see any of his grandchildren. Maybe the war and the stress he suffered while incarcerated behind barbed wire got the best of him for he died about 10 years thereafter of a heart attack at the age of 58.

It was good to get back to Oslo again even though I missed my family and friends up north. Here in my old neighborhood, I had my old friends and soon made new ones. The midnight sun does not shine as far south as Oslo, but during the summer months there is plenty of daylight late into the evening. My old friends and I had lots of time to get reacquainted with each other and roam around exploring the city. Trips down to the docks were always very exciting because there were always strange new things to see there. One day we had an unusual find; there were bits of copra (industrial grade coconut) and small pieces of black licorice strewn throughout the area. During the unloading, small pieces of copra had fallen from the clamshell bucket that was used to unload the ships. We were told that copra was one of the ingredients used in the manufacturing of soap and licorice was used in the making of tobacco products. Since neither I nor my friends could ever remember seeing or even tasting copra or licorice before, this was an interesting find and started a life-long fondness for licorice.

On my last trip to the waterfront, I was surprised to see a large rusty ship covered with barnacles tied up at the dock. The ship turned out to be the German ship *S/S Donau* that was destroyed during the war by the resistance using Limpet mines. The ship was used by the German military to transport troops, equipment, war supplies and, at times, prisoners between Norway and northern Europe. The ship had been re floated a few weeks earlier and was now on the way to the scrap yard to be dismantled. Before it could leave, the ship had to be emptied and somewhat cleaned up. Besides all the rust and barnacles covering the ship there was a huge dent at the stern. The dent must have been the impact point when the ship hit the rocky bottom during the attempted beaching. I don't remember seeing the holes made by the exploding Limpet mines. I suppose those holes had already been repaired in order to keep the ship afloat. I have had a difficult time over the years to forget the rusted cars, barnacles, war equipment, piles of horse skeletons and bones sticking out of the mud that were being hoisted out of the ship's cargo hold and loaded onto railroad cars for shipment to the dump. The smell of all that rotten cargo was very strong and lingered around for a long time.

Chapter 5

I was now in the early stages of becoming a young adult and it was time for me to think about the future. I was still in mandatory public school, but in my spare time, I would work for the telephone company delivering telegrams. When I had a little extra free time and money, I would sign up and take night classes. Some of the subjects that fascinated me were oil painting and history. I knew that there was no chance of ever making a living at any of the things that I enjoyed as a hobby, but it didn't matter. Those were very exciting times in my life; so many good things were happening all at once.

By now I was out of grade school and had just finished my second year of middle school studying machine works, mechanical drawing and such. I was thinking that I might like to work in the engine room on ships as a marine engineer. There was a demand for sailors at that time but it was also very common for young boys in Norway to go to sea, hopefully to mature and also to see a little of the outside world.

I signed with a Norwegian shipping company and was assigned as an engine boy to a ship named *M/S Black Condor*. The company provided me with airfare from Oslo to Amsterdam, Holland and by bus to Rotterdam where the ship was docked. It was very exciting to me. I got to fly to a foreign country and have a real job with a paycheck. My job in the engine room didn't turn out the way I expected; there was no training, just a lot of cleaning. We cleaned and painted all day long, from sunrise to sunset, it seemed. But it wasn't all bad; I was furnished board and room and got to travel for free and learn a little about the world. Our first port of call was Bremen, Germany. After we docked and I went on deck, it was as if someone had hit me in the face. There was total destruction everywhere I looked. I didn't see one complete building standing in any direction, just piles upon piles of bricks. There were longshoremen everywhere working our winches unloading and loading the ship. Every so often, one of them would walk by me and whisper in broken English asking if I had any cigarettes he could buy from me. I had none, I didn't smoke.

I was a total greenhorn and had no idea about what was going on. We were to stay in Bremen for a couple days so I asked one of my shipmates who wanted to sightsee if it would be okay if I tagged along with him. We took a cab to the main part of the city and everywhere I looked there were piles of bricks, some as high as two or three story buildings. But, when I looked closely I could see openings here and there. Behind the openings under all that rubble I saw lights and people, shops and all types of establishments. I could not believe my eyes. Our next stop was Hamburg where we went through the same routine at the dock, longshoremen everywhere asking for cigarettes. I soon found out that the price for a carton of cigarettes was 1 dollar. Our price was only 85 cents per carton while we were in international waters. But I hadn't been in international waters yet so I had to be satisfied just watching all the others trading. What was left of this beautiful city,

Hamburg, was pretty much the same as Bremen—piles upon piles of bricks. I could see nothing of value standing in any direction. We again took a cab into the city where we were faced with the same sight as Bremen, just rubble. We stopped at a very nice restaurant underneath the rubble and my friend ordered schnapps. To my surprise, I was served too although I was way under age, which didn't seem to matter. I was not used to alcohol so I declined anymore after the first one. When we got back to the ship from our excursion, we were bombarded with questions from some of the other shipmates who were all in various stages of intoxication. The main talk was about women, prostitution and how much money things cost.

But soon we were on our way again to our next stop, which was New York City. A few days into the Atlantic Ocean we ran into bad weather. I was amazed to see waves as tall as small buildings tossing our big ship around like a toy boat. Everything was tied down and the wind was so strong that it was difficult to walk across the deck. I was seasick for about four days but I didn't miss any work since being seasick was something that I should expect until I found my sea legs.

Arriving in New York was very exciting; Times Square, The Empire State Building, Rockefeller Center, it was all here and I just didn't feel that I had seen enough of it before we left. Our next stop was Boston, then Baltimore, Philadelphia and Norfolk. While in Norfolk, I took time off and went on a sightseeing bus trip to Washington D.C. It turned out to be one of the most interesting things that I had ever done. We had access to and got to see just about all the main places for which the city is famous, including President Truman's Oval Office.

Then we went back to New York for more cargo and again headed back out into the Atlantic Ocean and the European Continent. I made six crossings like that before I decided that a sailor's life was lonely, uncertain and not for me. Arriving back to Oslo was very interesting. When I left, my friends were all young adults; now they were grownups with jobs and some even in relationships. I got a job nearby and went back to night school, still wondering what was next for me. I still enjoyed traveling, history and investigating new places. So one day when my buddy asked me if I could get off work and could afford to join him and a number of other people on a bus excursion from Oslo to the French Riviera and back, I was very pleased. That sounded like something that would be lots of fun as well as educational. The trip was phenomenal, lots of sightseeing and full of ancient as well as recent history.

Chapter 6

When I got back home my mother told me that she had been in contact with her family in America. They had told her that they would sponsor us if we wanted to come. It was a time when the political forecast between the East and West was not good and was getting worse each day. The Korean conflict was not going well for the West and threats of outright global war were on the horizon. Our thoughts were that since we had been living in a war-torn country through one world war that was enough. My mother made arrangements to put some distance between us and the threats from the Eastern Bloc.

We had family in both Montana and Washington State who were willing to sponsor us. But there was lots of paperwork ahead before we could even apply for a visa. The U.S. Embassy wanted proof that we were worthy of coming to America. We had to provide them with official signed papers from the Health Department that we were sane and had never been hospitalized for insanity, never have had syphilis and presently did not have a venereal disease. From the Police Department, a statement that we never had been incarcerated or arrested for a serious crime and that we didn't owe any taxes. Since the American dollars were in short supply in Norway at that time, we were only allowed to exchange and take no more than seventy-five dollars per person out of the country. We were also informed that when we arrived in America we were not to replace or take work away from any legal U.S. citizen. Since we didn't have money for all of us to travel together, my mother decided that I should go first. I could then write back and explain to her what my reception was like. Eventually all the paperwork came together and I was on my way as a passenger onboard the *S/S Stavangerfjord* to a new life in America. The bus trip from New York City to Montana took three days.

I spoke very little English and never knew how long we would be at each stop so I would hurry and buy an apple as that was one of the words I knew. When I arrived in Montana, I felt totally out of my element — geographically as well as socially. It was a beautiful place, high mountains and wide-open spaces, just very nice. When the wind blew I saw tumbleweeds tumbling across the prairie and I thought this was the real Wild West. I could hardly believe my eyes that I was really here. A few times when I saw cowboys rounding up cattle, I thought the only thing missing was to see John Wayne on his horse coming over the hill. My transition into this new lifestyle was relatively easy. I wanted to be part of it and tried very hard to fit in as quickly as possible. I made friends easily and had a few jobs that paid very well. The best paying job I had (about 25 dollars a day) was working with a 14-men sheep shearing crew traveling from ranch to ranch.

My job consisted of getting into an 8-foot long burlap sack, 4-feet in diameter, which was suspended through a hole from a 9-foot high scaffold. After the wool was clipped and tied, it was then thrown into the sack that I was in. I was to walk around compressing as much of the wool as possible. When I eventually stomped myself out of the sack (about 32 to 34 pieces later), I would motion to one of the other fellows below to help me raise the sack so I could sew it together at the top. I would then let go of the sack, put a new one in the hold and start all over again. The only drawback to the job was that after each shift my clothing was almost completely stiff and covered in lanolin, sheep feces and ticks.

The other jobs I had were much more pleasant but paid a lot less and for awhile I worked for only board and room. It didn't take me long before I realized that good language skills were necessary in order to fit in and obtain a good job. Since I was a legal resident of military age, it wasn't long before the Selective Service contacted me to sign up with them. They explained that since I was not a U.S. Citizen yet, I could not be drafted unless I waived that right.

A few months went by and the next thing I knew I was on my way to Fort Ord, California for basic training. The training consisted of discipline, getting us in good physical shape, explaining military code and introducing us to all the weapons available to the infantry, as well as how to handle live ammunition. The second phase of my training took place at Fort McClellan, Alabama, where we were trained in CBR (Chemical, Biological, Radiological) warfare. Some of our training was in how to use a Geiger counter. We all wore name tags that were made out of lead and were backed by unexposed film. After each field trip, we had to turn in our name tags to have the film developed. If our name was readable on the film, that meant that we had been exposed to a high dose of radiation that day. The rumor was that we were being trained to take part in the atomic bomb testing in the Nevada desert.

Wearing Uncle Sam's uniform and serving in the U.S. Army Chemical Corps was very interesting, but not always without surprises. One morning after roll call, I heard my name and several other names called out. The rest of the troops were dismissed. As I stood there in place, totally confused, our First-Sergeant walked over toward us and said, "It has come to the attention of the Army that none of you are U.S. Citizens. You people are not supposed to be here. A mistake has been made so to rectify the mistake, the Army will take you to the Federal District Court in Birmingham, Alabama and petition the Court to grant you U.S. Citizenship as soon as possible. Those of you who want to become U.S. Citizens, report to the Provost Marshal's office in one hour wearing your Class-A uniform. The Provost Marshal will provide transportation and will personally drive you to the courthouse."

A few weeks later we all returned to the courthouse and became US. Citizens. For whatever reason, it really improved my self-esteem. I no longer felt like an outsider. I became acquainted with a lot of fellows like myself during the training and I suppose we all felt like most young boys at that age: totally indestructible. Some of those fellows got assigned to the same overseas unit as I did and we became lifelong friends. Others were assigned to companies in Korea and the rest went to the atomic testing grounds in Nevada. Being part of such a mixture of different people, cultures and religions was a totally new experience to me. It was an eye-opener. I must have lived a very sheltered life as a youngster. I loved listening to some of the more outspoken and experienced recruits when they told stories during our free times and in the barracks. The stories were generally about girlfriends but sometimes also of scary and supernatural events. I was too inexperienced for telling stories myself and too embarrassed to tell stories from my childhood since the only scary stories I was familiar with were stories where trolls were the main characters.

Walter Willanger

Chapter 7

A troll is a fictional character from Norway. Trolls come in a variety of sizes from very small to huge. They are extremely ugly, have bulging eyes, a long nose and a tail. Some live in the forests and others live in the mountains. As I got older, many other types of trolls were introduced into my reading vocabulary. They were all very scary. But not until I was a teenager did ghosts and demons and the supernatural enter my psyche. I remember being told by my elders that I must always respect the dead. I was told that they were angels in heaven and they keep an eye on things here on earth. One of the worst things one could do was to purposely step or walk on a dead person's grave, disturb the headstone, steal flowers from their grave, or just disrespect their resting place. If you did violate these rules, then they would come and pay you a visit in the night. So, if you awoke in the morning with a blue-colored bruise on your body, that meant that you had been visited and pinched by a dead person's ghost. It was all very confusing to me as a young boy, thinking that when people died they became angels, ghosts, evil spirits, and all sorts of strange things, maybe even reincarnated.

So while listening to my fellow recruits, I now realized that there must be thousands of different religions, beliefs, folklore and supernatural events buried in past history as well as new ones coming to light each day. As I think back, so much of the folklore throughout the world consists of a constant struggle between angels and devils, good and evil, light and dark and daytime and night time. Many societies live and die and some survive on information passed from generation to generation and could possibly self-destruct if those chains were broken. It's a very strong belief system.

Chapter 8

As a soldier, I traveled to many places within the United States but eventually got stationed permanently at Mildenhall Air Force Base in England, a few miles outside of London. Our company was there to support the Air Force as well as to hide the airfield with smoke in case we were attacked by low-flying hostile aircraft. In my spare time, I volunteered and became part of the Army Drill Team, going from town to town presenting the colors and promoting goodwill. When my tour of duty came to an end, I was shipped to Fort Sheridan, Illinois and discharged. I was paid traveling expenses back to Montana from where I was drafted. But to find a good paying job there other than ranching would be difficult. By now I was spoiled and was interested in finding a more challenging job, preferably in the industrial sector.

I was encouraged by some of the fellows at the Veterans Administration to go back to school and learn something about the many newly developed fields in areas such as industrial electronics. I then asked a number of people in the area what they knew about electricity and if they had any idea of how television worked. The answer I most often got was, "I stay away from anything that has to do with electricity." This was a very strange answer, I thought, so if I chose electronics for a living, I certainly would not have as much competition as in other fields. I decided then to travel to Seattle, Washington where I found a technical school that was teaching basic and advanced electronics, but they had a waiting list. While waiting for acceptance, I gathered all my school records from Norway and the Army and forwarded them to the School Board who told me what subjects I needed to complete in order to get a high school diploma here. Going to high school full time and working was not easy but necessary. About two years later came the very proud moment in my life. I had graduated along with many other very young high school students.

I went back to the technical school and was immediately enrolled. Electronics turned out to be very complicated and complex. I was learning words and things that I had never heard before. Each day was painful and full of demanding assignments. It was an uphill battle for me. Through school I had become acquainted with a number of people, both male and female, and it was through one of them that I met my future wife, Myrna. Looking back, I don't think I was a very exciting date, since many of our dates consisted of her reading from the FCC License Q&A manual and asking me questions that I had to learn the answers to, or else she would be looking through my lesson plan and ask me questions that I knew my instructor would test me on.

As time went by, I got more and more confident in myself as well as in the curriculum that I had chosen. My personal relationship with Myrna was good but not without problems. Her family roots were Irish, Dutch and German. I was foreign born and of a different religion. This was a big problem in those days but we got used to it and without anyone's blessings proceeded to get married.

A few months into our marriage we had a daughter. It was very scary to be a father with so much responsibility. I quit school before graduation and was lucky enough to get a job at the Boeing Company in numerical control, a newly developed field. It was wonderful to have a job with a real future. We could now buy groceries, baby food and even indulge in a little luxury.

Our second child was a boy. He was born too early and passed away shortly after delivery. This was very painful for both of us but when I saw my wife at the maternity ward, I could tell that she was extremely depressed. I don't think she ever got over it. Eventually we had two more children, both daughters. I loved my three daughters more than I ever thought would be possible. Just seeing and hearing them play was like music to my ears. Our finances were pretty meager but we lived a pretty normal life entertaining ourselves by going on overnight camping trips, taking the girls to the drive-in movie theaters, playing games at home and just enjoying each other.

About 15 years into the marriage, the many internal and external problems that my wife and I started out with in the very beginning began to take their toll. We stayed together for another 10 years but when the last child moved out of our home, the marriage dissolved. Starting a new life by myself was not easy but it was better than living in a stressful relationship. After the divorce, my ex-wife and I had a few friendly meetings with regard to questions about the children. But all that came to an end one dark night when she was killed in a car accident.

Chapter 9

I was not interested in a new relationship until I met Dolores. Over the years I had seen her with her husband at a couple of functions that my wife and I also attended, but we were never introduced. One day I had to go to downtown Seattle to see an attorney regarding some business. Little did I know that she worked nearby. It was very comforting for me to see and talk with her since she was a person who I barely knew and she was not in a position to take sides about my divorce.

I then mustered up some courage and asked her if I could join her for a cup of coffee during her break. From the conversation we had, I found out that she had been divorced for 3 years, she had a 9-year old son at home and she was also taking care of her elderly, widowed father who was living with her. I thought she was very cheerful even carrying such responsibilities. Her interests were in books, art, and many of the things that I enjoyed, plus she was a wonderful and articulate conversationalist. Cautiously, I asked her if she, in the future sometime, would like to meet me again for coffee, lunch, or even take in a movie. As time went by, we had several dates and I was introduced to her father and her youngest son. She met my daughters and the other family members. We took things somewhat slowly at the beginning since we both were a little gun shy about getting into a new, serious relationship. Throughout the following year, I met her other grown boys as well as her sister and her other family members whom I enjoyed very much.

Besides painting with oil on canvas, I had another hobby which was making family film journals. I had also produced several TV commercials which were aired in the Seattle area, made a medical teaching film and a couple short-subject children's fairy tales.

My next project was to spend my vacation traveling throughout the South Pacific filming the journey of Captain Cook and showing how the places he visited looked now. Loaded down with camera equipment and 16mm movie film, Dolores and I and another filmmaker traveled to Australia where we had signed on as guest-crew on one of the world's few remaining square-rigged sailing ships, *The Eye of the Wind*. We sailed Australia's Great Barrier Reef to such remote places as Raine Island, Cook Town, Endeavor Reef, and Cape York, filming all the time.

This was a life-changing experience for us. With the exception of now having modern, up-to-date maps and navigation equipment, we lived like the sailors did years ago. We stood watches around the clock, pulled and set sails and kept the ship in good, clean order. Our air conditioner below deck consisted of a couple of canvas tubes that were strung from above deck through a walkway channeling the air to the interior of the ship. If the wind was strong the air conditioner worked good, but usually it was too hot to sleep below deck during the day. Several of the crew who worked the night watch then would take naps on the windy and shady side on the deck. The guest-crew was not expected to climb the riggings but in order for me to get the right film shot, they allowed me to do it. Climbing the mast was scary, especially going from one section of the mast, crawling under the platform onto the top of the platform where the new mast section started. For me, setting and taking in the sails was the hardest since my hands were not calloused and the ropes (lines) felt like pulling on sandpaper. I have to give credit to all our predecessors who sailed these ships years ago. They did a good job without much complaining.

Our land excursions were always exciting because we visited places that could only be reached by ship. Some had never been visited before and others that hadn't been visited by people for years. Each time we went ashore on a remote, uninhabited beach to explore something of historical nature, the first-mate would caution us about picking things up.

There are many things to be aware of in the warm, tropical waters such as cone shells (Conidea) which are home to predatory sea snails. These snails are equipped with a very venomous harpoon enabling them to catch and kill prey quickly and will also harpoon people if one gets too close. Another creature we should stay away from was a very small, blue-ringed octopus that with its bite can inject enough poison to kill a person within a very few minutes. Australia's Raine Island was another place of extreme interest. The island is a bird sanctuary and one of the few places that is inhabited by the green turtle. We arrived during the egg-laying season and were lucky enough to witness from a distance hundreds of turtles laying their eggs. The island is also the place where a stone beacon, the oldest European structure in the Australian tropics, is located. The beacon was built in 1844 by the British Admiralty using prison labor.

Just off shore are the remains of more than thirty shipwrecks which include the HMS Pandora. The ship was lost on her return voyage to England with some of the HMS Bounty mutineers who were captured in Tahiti and were now to be returned to England to stand trial. Sailing for a day with a good breeze behind, we located a pearling station. Behind the primitive dock was a very pretty, long, sandy beach. It was decided that we should drop anchor here and check it out. On shore we were met by an Islander named Ben. He told us that this was a blister pearl station that was no longer in use. He carried a shotgun and a long spear and was the only person living on the island. Since there wasn't much going on there, the owners had asked him if he would keep an eye on the place.

I was sure he didn't have many visitors through the years, so I asked him about the gun and the spear. He said that the gun was for the snakes and the spear was for the salt-water crocodiles. I then asked him if he had seen any crocodiles nearby lately, to which he answered yes. We had fresh fish onboard so our captain asked Ben if we could use his beach and if he would join us in a fish fry. I asked Dolores to sit next to Ben and I would sit next to her. I said to her, "If Ben gets up in a hurry and starts running, remember to get up and we will run as fast as we can after him. We just have to trust his judgment." Anyway, we had no unexpected creature visitors during our fish fry and it all turned out fine. This whole trip was turning out to be like an adventure story and it had just started.

A few years later, we made room for another unforgettable trip. My fascination with art, especially oil paintings from the 17th through the 19th centuries, really held my interest. We decided to start our travel in the Provence region of France.

I had read that one of the old masters had said that the light there was so perfect to paint by. On our way to Paul Cezanne's home town, Aix-En-Provence, we drove past a small village where we decided to take a break. In the village square stood an unusual looking church, the Basilica of St. Maximin. This was something that we had not planned on but was a total bonus for us. The church dates back to the mid-1200s and it is still used for worship. Below ground level, we went to a crypt that holds the skull that has long been worshipped as that of St. Mary Magdalene. I was totally overcome and could hardly believe that I was standing there looking and being in the presence of such holiness. This was biblical history. We took some photos of the church and its interior and continued on our way.

There are a lot of memorials to Paul Cezanne's life in Aix-En-Provence, including the house where he was born, his work studio and the house where he lived as an adult and later died. On our way to Arles, about an hours' drive away, we passed through the town of Salon-de-Provence. It was here that Nostradamus lived and wrote many of his quatrains and prophesies. The house where he spent the last few years of his life has been made into a museum. He died here and was buried in town but was later reburied in the wall of the church Collegiale Saint-Laurent.

The following day, we made our way to the town of Arles. While Vincent Van Gogh lived in this town, he created many of his now famous paintings such as *Pavement Café at Night*, *The Yellow House*, and many others. It was also in the yellow house during a drunken episode with Paul Gauguin that he got so mad and despondent that he cut off his ear lobe. As a result, he personally had himself admitted for treatment at Saint-Remy's hospital for the mentally ill, a short distance from Arles. During his stay at the hospital, he was allowed to paint since painting was very therapeutic for him. Part of the hospital is now a museum and open to the public. There were reproductions of his paintings throughout the property. The reproductions were located at the exact places he stood while painting each painting. Upon his release from the hospital, he was encouraged to move away and get a new, fresh start somewhere else. He chose a little village north of Paris by the name Auvers-sur-Oise.

He continued to paint but his mental state was far from cured. Whatever demons he was struggling to control continued to bother him. The rumor is that one day while he was out in the field painting, he decided to end it all. He pulled out a revolver, shot himself in the chest and died three days later. New information suggests that he might have been shot accidently by two young boys from the village who were playing with a revolver. We went to the cemetery where we found his grave and were glad to see that it was still very well maintained after all these years. So many of the great painters, writers and composers from that era had such an unappreciated end to their life, it just didn't seem fair to me.

As our time overseas was coming to an end, we had to travel through Bavaria, Germany for our flight back home. In doing so, we would be traveling through the town of Neuschwanstein, where King Ludwig's fairytale castle is located. Being such a popular site for visitors from all over the world, we were very lucky to go through the castle without much waiting. Another village about an hour away from the castle was the town of Berchtesgaden. It is here, high in the mountains, that Hitler's Eagle's Nest is located. Since there wasn't a cloud in the sky, we thought the view from there would be fantastic.

From a collection point, we walked through a tunnel into the mountain, then took an elevator that had been blasted all the way to the top. When the elevator doors opened, we were actually inside the Eagle's Nest. The view in every direction was impressive. In the main conference room, there was a film from 1945 showing American soldiers inspecting the Eagle's Nest. Since I lived through that era and was now seeing films and pictures from that time, it brought back some unpleasant memories of the German occupation. It also made me uneasy walking around in the same space that so many of the decision makers had walked while making decisions that caused so much death and hell for much of the world. It's all part of history now and I must say I really enjoyed the rest of Bavaria which is a beautiful, scenic part of the world.

Our relationship was very comfortable and we had a relaxing and fun time together. So after some time, Dolores and I decided to get married. The wedding was a private affair that included only our children, family and a few close friends.

Walter Willanger

Chapter 10

Have you ever wondered how it feels to die? One minute you are alive and vibrant, talking and making decisions. Then, in the blink of the eye, it's all gone. You are now just a dead body. Hopefully you are one of the lucky ones and someone will have started CPR on you. If not, seconds is all you have and then your organs will start to fail, one by one. As time ticks away, you get closer and closer to eternity from which there is no return.

In the early hours of October 1, 2006, it happened to me. My heart stopped (sudden cardiac arrest). I was dead for 1 hour and 14 minutes. As of this printing, I'm still among the living. How can that be? Was it a miracle? Medical intervention? Or just luck?

Since that time, I have been approached by acquaintances and strangers, as well as other heart patients who have heard of this incident and who have asked me to tell them what happened to me. Initially, I never put much thought into their questions because I felt there wasn't very much to tell. It was over in the blink of an eye.

Then one day, my wife asked me to go with her to a show where one of this nation's most famous psychics was to perform. I told her yes, I would like to go, thinking it would be an interesting event. Maybe the psychic could shed some light on some of the things that I experienced during and after my sudden death event. This psychic has in the past helped solve a number of unsolved disappearances and mysteries for the police. We arrived to a totally packed theater and were given numbered tickets. We were told to guard the ticket stubs because later during the show a few numbers would be called out and the person who had the ticket stub with that number would be allowed to ask the psychic one question.

To our surprise, my number was called. I had not prepared myself for this. What should I ask? Then suddenly, it was my turn in front of this large audience. With microphone in hand, I said, "A while back I had a heart attack, my heart stopped." I hadn't finished the sentence before the psychic answered me…"You must write a book about it."

Chapter 11

Upon leaving the theater, I was surprised by how many people from the audience approached me and bombarded me with questions such as, "My friend's heart stopped, they used an electrical defibrillator and CPR on him but he died anyway. Do you think he suffered?" Then others asked, "What was it like for you?" "Did you see anything?" "How do you feel now?" and many more questions.

After months of consideration, I decided that I should be writing a book about my sudden death experience. I was thinking that putting my experience in writing could be helpful to me as well as to people who have had loved ones pass over to the other side and were still wondering whether the passage was peaceful or not. For centuries, people have been fascinated with death and dying. It is a subject I know many of us have been touched by.

Most of the old European religious doctrines are based on what will happen to us after we die or in life hereafter. Some suggest that we continue to live in spirit form forever and we will be rewarded in heaven if we lived a good life here on earth. The other choice is going to hell where one will live in fire for eternity. From what I have observed, Eastern religions and beliefs seem to be more about living a good life now and teaching people the importance of knowledge, peace and loving each other while we are still here on earth. Have we outgrown the old-fashioned belief, "Do unto others as you want others to do unto you."? But, whatever religious beliefs one has are his or her business and are not the subject of this writing.

Chapter 12

Throughout the world there are celebrations where we include the dead. In Mexico, they have a yearly celebration Day of the Dead or Dia de los Muertos. On my first trip to Mexico, I was totally surprised to see all the wooden and ceramic skeletons and skulls for sale at the market place and

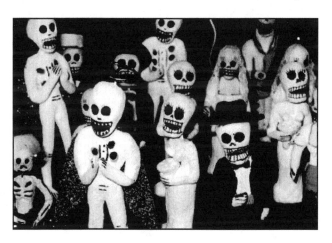

Day of the Dead Celebration

in so many of the places that cater to tourists. I didn't know much about the celebration at that time but I now understand that it is a way to honor and to keep in touch with the departed. The celebrations are as if the dead are still among us and on a particular date in the autumn, they celebrate the spirits' returning. They then offer the spirits food and a lot of attention.

South America, Africa and many Asian nations have also set aside dates to honor and celebrate the dead.

My Chinese friend told me that where he came from, they had two funerals. The first one was shortly after death when the body was buried in the ground. The second funeral was the following year when the bones were dug up, washed with wine or special liquid and placed in a large crock above the ground. I was told that this was partially due to a shortage of permanent burial space.

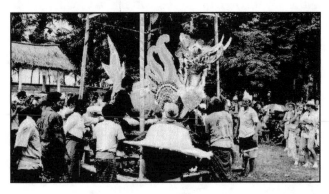

Cremation Ritual in Bali

On the island of Bali, Indonesia, they keep the body of the departed at home until they have enough money for a proper funeral. At that time, the body arrives in an elaborately decorated papier-mache casket carried on top of a tall wooden structure by their friends. As the procession walks toward the cremation place, the casket is turned around and around in circles to confuse the spirit. At the chosen place, the casket is placed onto a pyre of wood and the deceased's oldest child has the honor of lighting the fire to cremate the remains and release the spirit into the afterworld. The Buddhists celebrate Obon to honor their departed ancestors and in Northern Europe, Canada and the United States, they celebrate Halloween.

The name Halloween and the tradition have been modified many times over the past several hundred years. It started out as a medieval festival of the dead, but throughout the ages, it has changed and is now more of a fun festival where trick or treat is the main theme. These are just a few examples of how differently some of our societies celebrate the very same thing. But, they all have one thing in common and that is to keep the communication open between the living and the dead.

Chapter 13

After my brief experience being among the dead, I find that I have more questions about death and dying than answers. Some people believe the dead have special powers and connections and that the dead can do us favors. Most of us celebrate and talk about the dead because we miss them and we have accepted the fact that we can never again spend time with them in this world. But, I think the real reason why we are fascinated with death and dying is because most people are afraid of dying. They are unsure and don't know what is waiting for them over on the other side.

We have been told and instructed that if we behave in a certain way, we will be rewarded after death. This is all very nice, but how do we know that we have been following the right religion or that we have behaved correctly? Not until the last few decades has the medical community been able to bring people who were clinically dead back to life. For the few of us who have experienced death, at least for a short while, and were lucky enough to be brought back to life, we all have experienced different things and the outcome of our experience was not always what we hoped for or expected.

Chapter 14

I talked earlier about my time with my grandmother who was born in 1864. She would tell and teach me about what it was like to be young during the 1800 era. My grandmother read the Bible all the time. It probably wasn't all the time but, to a young boy, once a day or so would seem to be very often. I think she felt that she understood the Bible because she was loving and understanding to all people she met.

For years I assumed she was a member of the Lutheran religion. But, recently I was told by a very trusted family member that the religion she practiced was an offshoot of a very old religion. Some people referred to her religion as a strange, outdated cult. But, at the very end, it doesn't matter whether we are members of a cult or of a mainstream religion so long as we conduct ourselves and try to live a good life according to whichever holy book we read. If we do this, we too will be remembered by our neighbors as a very kind and good person.

Not very far from my grandmother's house lived my aunt, uncle and cousin who was just a couple years older than me. I was a boy under the age of 10 years when my cousin died. He was very sick the last time I saw him, and at that time he asked me, "Are you afraid of me?"

"No," I said, which was a lie. Of course I was afraid of him. I was also afraid of catching whatever he had. For months after the funeral when we visited my aunt and uncle's home, my imagination would go into high alert. I remember one night our family stayed overnight at their home. All I could think of was the funeral and ghosts and each creak or squeak I heard was in my mind some ghosts trying to alert me of things to come. I don't think I slept the whole night. Even though I had to go to the bathroom, I lay and waited until someone else had to go and allowed me to go along.

The biggest shock of my life came the day my mother died. She had been ill for awhile but I didn't know that it was serious. We had for years had a very good relationship and talked about everything between heaven and earth, except for her illness. This she kept private. I suppose she didn't want to worry anyone. My mother was very well-read and would talk to me about some of the things she had read. We would share stories and laugh; other times we would disagree. I think we covered just about every subject under the sun.

One day she wanted to tell me a story she had read about two people who had made a pact. They had promised each other that whoever died first would, if it was possible, come back and tell the other what it was like over on the other side.

Curious, I asked my mother if that was something that she had read or if this was something she had done? After a few denials, she admitted to me that she and her mother had made that pact. Her mother had died several years before I was born and I was now an adult. Obviously I wanted to know whether she was ever contacted by her mother over the years. My curiosity was killing me. Then finally she admitted to me that she wasn't sure. Whatever it was that she thought was a contact turned out to be bogus. I then told her that I wanted to make contact with her after she or I died.

At first she said that she didn't want to. "Why?" I would ask her.

"Because, if I come back you will get so scared that it will cause you to have a heart attack and that I don't want to be responsible for," she told me. Shortly thereafter came the very saddest day. I was informed that my mother had passed away during the night. I had a very difficult time accepting that, and the fact that we no longer belonged in the same environment was troubling. We were totally separate now. It was a strange feeling. The last thing she said to me as she was going to bed was, "There is something that I want to tell you but I can't remember. I will tell you tomorrow." There was no tomorrow. But, there was much more to talk about and things to enjoy and it all now came to a screeching halt. The very difficult mourning period seemed to last forever but, as time and years passed, it got better.

Chapter 15

I think that when we finally accept our loss and we rethink our relationship and rebuild our memories, it gets better. I never again thought about some of the strange things that my mother and I talked about until one afternoon. I had just returned home from work and I was very tired. I decided to take a nap. As I was drifting off into a dream-like slumber, I heard my mother calling out to me. Then she told me that she had seen this person that we both knew who had just recently died, but she had not talked to her yet. Then again she called out to me as if she wanted my full attention: "Walter!" This time so loud that I jumped out of bed wide awake. I sat there on the edge of the bed for a minute wondering whether I was hallucinating or going crazy. Never again did an episode like that happen, even years later while I was on the other side and we had no barrier between us. That was disappointing to me because if she could have made contact with me, she could have at that time. It is strange what the brain is able to do to us to protect us if necessary.

I know a lady who told me about what happened to her when she was a ten-year old girl. She had been outside her house playing with her friends and decided to take a break.

As she entered the house, she found her mother lying on the floor dead. What a shock. The mother had died very quickly from heart failure. In those days, few people knew of such a thing as a support group or any other type of professional counseling for such a traumatic event. In order for this young girl to survive the pain and trauma and live a normal life, over time, she developed a mental block as to her mother. To this day, she cannot remember her times with her mother even though she was the apple of her mother's eye and they were physically and emotionally never very far apart from each other. When she tries to call up memories of her mother, she always sees her mother lying face-up on the kitchen floor and that is all. All other images of their relationship have been erased.

Our mind is capable of so many things such as denial, remembrance, trickery, as well as suggestions and many more. This story happened to my wife and me some time ago when we went on one of our many weekend trips. It was autumn, a beautiful crisp day in Oregon. We were driving along the coastal highway, just sightseeing. At that time of the year, most tourists have gone home and many places have closed for the winter ahead. We also didn't pay much attention to the time of day until the fog started to roll in. We were too far from home for us to turn around and drive back so we decided to find a place to spend the night. There were no vacancies in the motels nearby so we drove inland. We found a small, old motel that had a vacancy sign but looked more like something out of a horror story than a place to spend the night. Unfortunately, that was all that was available so we checked in. We had a very uneventful night until early morning. My wife woke up to the sound of someone knocking on the door. Who could that be? I went to investigate but saw no one. Then, the knocking started again; this time closer to the windows, higher and much louder. This went on for a long time, back and forth, up and down. It was driving us crazy. Is the motel possessed and full of demons? We couldn't get out of the motel fast enough. We gathered our stuff and made sure that all was clear and ran out as fast as we could. We got into the car and shut the doors. Just then something went by us in a hurry and landed in a tree next to the car. We both started to laugh, our nightmare turned out to be a woodpecker. We created our own nightmare. The sounds we heard was him pecking on the wall and the rest was our imagination.

Yes, the brain is very powerful and can serve us in all types of situations, both good and bad. All the different types of supernatural stories that I heard when I was very young must have made quite an impression on me. The stories made me very inquisitive but also frightened me a lot.

One story in particular that I remember was of a fellow in our village who was also a close neighbor. He worked part-time as the village gravedigger. At that time, the village was small and the gravedigger would not be very busy. I overheard him telling another man that he was always notified by the dead person when it was time for him to go to work. He continued by telling him that he would hear very light but persistent tapping on his bedroom window and that was the signal for him to go to the cemetery and get things in order and start digging. I was surprised at that story because his hearing was very bad and he said the tapping was light.

I was sure he was telling the truth; he was an adult and adults didn't lie to each other. Maybe he knew I was listening and his intention was to scare me and if so, he did a good job. As I told this story to my friends, they would tell me similar stories of small birds tapping on the windows of people to notify the resident of impending death in the family. That really bothered me since I had seen birds tapping on windows very often and nothing ever happened. Finally, I made it my duty to spy on the birds to see what was going on. After some time, I spotted a couple of birds who were sitting on the window sill eagerly tapping, but not on the window. They were eating the putty that was there to keep the window pane in place. Although I had now solved one of the problems that had scared me as a child, the impact of these stories stayed with me for a lifetime.

Chapter 16

The good thing about hearing these stories is that they made me think and pay attention to detail. Although I missed or let go of the big picture once in awhile, I did zero in on what I considered to be important details. I have never been an exercise-type of a person but I do enjoy exercise in the form of walking. At home I would walk on the sidewalk next to the beach and at my place of employment I would park my car as far away from my work station as possible. That way I felt I had a little control of my body in areas such as weight gain or loss.

At that time in my life there was also a lot of talk and information about heart workout and getting the pulse rate at a particular point. I felt the amount of walking that I was doing was enough since I was keeping good track of how I felt. I remember one morning in the middle of winter, I had parked my car and had walked briskly in the cold air about three-quarters of a mile towards my work station. All of a sudden I was out of breath. This was unusual, I thought. I stopped and rested for a few minutes and then continued. This was a piece of detail that I must keep track of. I must remember and see if the same symptoms return the next time I walk.

The following morning the weather was a little warmer and I felt good with no shortage of breath during my walk. I then got thinking about what I had learned in biology class years ago, that our blood vessels are very sensitive to heat and cold. When the weather is cold, they contract a little in order to restrict the blood flow and keep the heat in next to the vital organs. My next question to myself was, could there already be some restrictions in my body due to plaque and cholesterol build up and the constrictions caused by the weather made me aware of it? During the following months, my routine was pretty much the same. Some days I would walk for miles and have no problems, while other days I was totally out of breath and could barely walk across the street. I was now paying more attention than ever before to details that my body was telling me.

At my next medical checkup, everything was fine until I mentioned this little detail to the doctor about how I had some problems catching my breath during cold weather walks.

"Oh, really? How long has that been going on?" he asked. He then took me by the arm and together we walked to the cardiologist at the clinic.

Chapter 17

My first brush with the idea that I might die took place several years ago. Until then, I was like most fellows, indestructible, and never thought about it. Death and dying were the last things on my mind. The whole chain of events started in the winter of 1992. Until that day, I was not aware of any health issues although I had noticed for awhile that when my body was under the slightest strain, my heart was working much harder than what I had been accustomed to. These symptoms did not come on overnight. Due to a stubborn streak of self-denial, almost a whole year went by before I made a decision to seek medical help for the problem that just wouldn't go away.

The checkup showed that I had cholesterol build-up (plaque) in several of the veins in the heart muscle. If untreated, a complete blockage would stop the blood flow to that particular part of the heart muscle and would cause the muscle to die. If that happened, then I would probably die immediately.

A medical procedure called angioplasty was suggested and scheduled. This procedure consisted of taking a thin wire with a small deflated balloon attached and inserting it into the artery in the groin and sliding it into the areas of blockage in the heart. When the balloon is in place, the balloon will be inflated and the blockage will be compressed so blood will flow freely again. My doctor explained to me that when the balloon is totally inflated, it is at that point that it will feel as if I were having a heart attack called coronary thrombosis. This procedure was performed on me but lasted only two months before the blockage was back. Then it was suggested that they try it again, which they did, but the second attempt lasted even less time.

Chapter 18

Then the unthinkable happened. I was taken by total surprise when I woke up in the early hours of June 26, 1994 and knew that something was wrong. I felt that I was in serious trouble due to a strange feeling in and around the heart. I jumped out of bed, grabbed my nitroglycerin pills, opened the bottle and took one. The strange feeling, which was a combination of pain and a heavy heart beat, stopped but did not go away. After about five minutes, I took another nitro pill; the result was the same. I instinctively knew that without medical support my life would be gone in a short time.

Although I'm not a very religious person, I became one immediately. I said a short prayer and asked for a little more time to live. If my prayer was granted, I vowed to help spread whatever information I had about heart disease to whoever would listen to me. That was a promise that I was going to keep. At the hospital, they did a complete checkup. The angiogram showed that I had a 98% blockage of the V. Cortdis Magna, commonly called the widow maker. A stent would be impossible due to the location of the blockage. There was only one option—immediate emergency by-pass surgery.

They placed me on a gurney and gave me a few minutes to get my personal things in order. I motioned for my wife to come closer; I wanted to tell her something. By now the sedative or tranquilizer that they had given me when I arrived at the hospital started to work. But what I wanted to tell my wife was that I loved her and that I would be right back as soon as the surgery was over. Instead, in my confused state of mind I asked her if she would please record a particular TV program for me in case I was still here in the afternoon. Because of the medication, I had no idea of the seriousness of the situation. I was then wheeled into a room where I saw a man dressed in green colored clothing, mask, headgear and arms crossed. Then everything went black.

At that time, I had a friend who was a retired Chief Petty Officer from the Coast Guard. To stay active in the community as well as to supplement his income, he went to work as a civilian contractor for various companies. His job was to conduct classes and show how OSHA could benefit the employees there. He told me years later that he had used me and the way that I behaved during my emergency as an example when he talked about attitude.

He told the story by saying that he had a friend who was in the hospital's emergency room being prepared to have major, emergency heart surgery. Not knowing whether he would survive the surgery or not, his family was gathered to say their last goodbyes. But, as he was being wheeled into the operating room, he said stop—he had something very important to say. The family in the waiting room held their breath thinking it must be his last wish or testament. No, all he wanted was to ask his wife to tape a particular TV program that he wanted to see. No one thought that he would survive the surgery except the patient himself. He expected to be back home in a few hours. Now that is a good attitude!

But, as I said before when I told the story, at that moment when I was being moved into surgery I was so relaxed and full of tranquilizers that my thinking was not up to standard. As I was coming out of the anesthesia a few hours later, I couldn't figure out how they could have hooked me up to all that equipment without me noticing it. Then someone asked me for my name and if I knew where I was. Only then did I realize that the surgery really was over.

Walter Willanger

Chapter 19

The following days went by without any major events. Upon being discharged from the hospital, I got a list of things not to do. The main thing was not to use my arms when I got up from a chair or out of bed. But for the first few weeks, I should also avoid pulling open or shutting doors, driving a car, vacuuming and everything else that would strain my chest muscles. After a few weeks at home, I returned again to the hospital for a post-operative checkup. I got a clean bill of health and at that time I got to meet the surgeon, a very pleasant man.

I recovered from the quadruple bypass surgery without any complications and felt very good physically. But, it was a very emotional and scary event and a tremendous wake-up call for me. From then on, I not only knew but understood that I was not invincible. I decided then that I must try to live the rest of my life to the fullest and no more wasting of time. Also high on the list was to spend as much time with my family and friends as I could. After all, your family could be all you have when it comes to your total support system.

I had a good job that I liked and that was fortunate. But I also wanted to continue my other dreams of visiting more places that I had read about, especially where historical and interesting events had taken place. As I wrote about earlier in this story, I was lucky enough to spend my vacation as a guest-crew member onboard a square-rigged sailing ship and sailed to places where Captain Cook and other earlier explorers left their marks.

But now, after my bypass surgery, I felt like damaged merchandise. For the time being, a trip such as that was now out of the question. I would not be able to perform some of the jobs that would be required of me. I had spent a lot of time as a young boy listening to my elders telling stories about life at sea and now the sea was off limits to me. I found this unacceptable but I soon found out that after months of healing there were still many places of interest left to visit where there is not such a medical risk factor involved. Life was great and I did all I could not to fall into the old trap of a hum-drum existence. Thinking back, I'm very happy about all the decisions that we made at that time.

We managed to travel to several of the remote, as well as to many of the more popular islands of the South Pacific. One of these journeys took us to Fiji. There weren't as many travelers visiting the islands of the South Pacific back then. The shortage of tourists was probably one of the reasons it was a little easier for us to make friends with the Islanders. A little over 150 years ago, not many of the people in the world knew much about the Fiji Islands other than that they were referred to as the Cannibal Islands. Fiji had no written language; their history was oral, passed from one generation to the next. After the mutiny on HMS Bounty, Captain Bligh and a number of his crew were set adrift in one of the ship's longboats and set course for Timor. He tried to avoid or not sail close to the unfriendly main islands of Fiji. But they did get so close to the nearby Yasawa island chain that they were spotted by the Islanders there. When they realized the Islanders were in hot pursuit after them, they took to the oars as well as the sails and each worked as hard as he could to distance themselves. Good thing they got away or history would have had a different ending.

We had a very interesting as well as a good time while we were in the Fiji Islands. One time my wife and I were invited by the village Chief to take part in an old-fashioned kava ceremony in the jungle after sunset. We had heard that kava was somewhat narcotic and to drink too much of it would make one lethargic and sleepy. In the old days, this type of ceremony was a serious and important affair. But now, it was just for show.

My wife and I arrived to a small opening in the jungle lit only by several small torches. When we arrived we were told to walk in a squatting manner. I was told to sit with my legs crossed and my wife with her legs to one side. At no time would anyone stand up or be taller than the Chief. We were sitting in a circle around the Tanoa (kava bowl). After everyone had arrived, one of the participants dipped the cup (half a coconut shell) in the bowl and passed it to me. I clapped twice, as instructed, and so did everyone else. I took the cup with both hands, took a sip and gave it back and clapped twice. The cup was then offered to the one sitting next to me and the same ritual followed. This went on for a long while until everyone in the circle had participated. In the past, this important ceremony was to show respect for authority, communal healing and the elders, etc.

Discipline for the average Fijian was stern. Any type of disrespect for the Chief, priest or any other high-ranking member of the tribe would be dealt with harshly, usually in death for the offender. Tribal warfare was also very common throughout the islands. The weapons were usually made from very hard ironwood. The main weapons used were two to three-foot long war clubs or shorter clubs with a big rugged ball on the end made for throwing. We were also told that as far as cannibalism was concerned, it was not just an act of getting something to eat, it was more ceremonial than anything else.

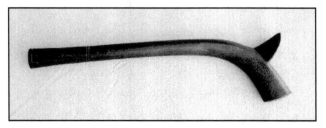

A Fijian War Club

I was told that after each battle, the warrior who fought best among the winners would get first choice. He would then pick among the dead enemies the one that he felt would be worthy of him. The thought was that by consuming his flesh, all the gallantry, bravery or whatever other assets the enemy possessed would be transferred to him. There was also a certain way the body was to be handled so as not to upset the energy. Different forks were used for each body part and to show the maximum amount of respect while consuming it; none of the flesh was to touch the outer part of one's lips.

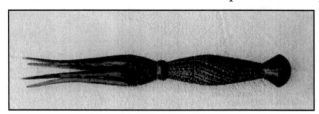

A Cannibal's Brain Fork

We experienced a number of informative and interesting things like that on each trip. For people with open minds, the world is a showcase of things to see and learn whether one is at home or far away. But as we know, reality sometimes has a surprising way of changing things. One morning I got the news that my only sibling, my sister, had suffered a heart attack. The day before, she had been complaining of having developed a cold and had tightness in the chest. She went to the neighborhood medical clinic to have it checked out. She explained to the doctor that there was a history of heart problems in the family and she wanted to know whether or not she was having a heart attack. That question could have been put to rest with a simple blood test. Without examining her, the doctor told her that it was probably a hiatal hernia giving her problems and she should go home and take a Pepcid antacid tablet; then she should be okay in the morning. Throughout the evening, she got worse and eventually went to the hospital emergency room.

Chapter 20

The diagnosis at the hospital was not good. She was indeed having a major heart attack and was admitted to the critical care unit barely alive. During the examination, it was discovered that there was a major blockage in her heart and the damage she had suffered was irreversible. If treatment had started at the time she first went to the medical clinic, there was a good chance that she would have been okay. At the hospital, she received the very best care and they tried everything to correct the damage including by-pass surgery. But, the damage that she sustained for not getting the correct medical diagnosis at the beginning was so extensive that she was dead within a year.

I feel there is a time when we should follow our gut instinct and be a little more demanding. My sister was like most people, she had total faith in the medical community and she paid for that with her life.

I enjoy talking and sharing stories with people. Some of these stories that I have heard are very good, others are just common everyday gossip. I particularly remember a very strange story that I would like to tell. I was walking next to the beach on a very nice afternoon when this man who was walking next to me started to talk and ask me questions. The fellow, I would guess, was in his mid-60s and spoke fluently and articulately but in broken English. His doctor had told him that he needed some exercise so he started to walk. Soon the conversation was about illnesses and he wanted to tell me about his experience leading up to his by-pass surgery. To make him feel better, I told him that I too have had by-pass surgery which he was not very interested in hearing about.

He continued by saying that one day while he was in the bathroom getting ready to go out, the next thing he remembered was his wife trying to wake him up. When he finally woke up, he asked his wife what happened. His wife told him that when she walked by the bathroom, she saw him lying on the bathroom floor with his head wedged between the stool and the bathtub. "You were sleeping so peacefully there that I let you sleep there for awhile."

He had received some bruises and a few cuts in the fall so 911 was called. The paramedics took care of the cuts and scrapes but upon further checking found out that he had passed out due to a small heart attack. At the hospital, they discovered that he also had severe coronary blockage and scheduled him for by-pass surgery.

He mentioned to me several times, "Why would anyone think I was taking a nap on the bathroom floor with my head between the stool and the bathtub?" I asked him if he and his wife had been arguing, or if they had been getting along? He told me that they had a perfect marriage and that all was fine with him and his wife as well as the children and grandchildren. Shortly thereafter, we parted company and I never saw him again. I have wondered many times what that was all about and what happened to him. I wondered why she delayed in calling 911 or seeking help for him. On my job and during my travels, I have met and talked to many fascinating people from all parts of the world. There seems to be something to be learned from each and every one of them but not always something productive.

Chapter 21

Some time ago, I was talking to a good friend of mine about sharing information about ourselves. He was very much against bothering people with his problems and illnesses. I told him that I was certainly glad for 911 and I knew of people who had been saved by their quick response. His answer was that he had lived long enough and what was good enough for his dad was good enough for him. He did not want anyone to call 911 and try to resuscitate him and that was spelled out in his Living Will, too.

One day while he was home alone watching TV, he started to feel a little lightheaded and had some chest discomfort. He got to the phone and dialed 911 so quickly it sounded like speed dialing. By now, he had changed his mind and wanted to live. If he had been unconscious when they got there and found his medical instructions (do not resuscitate), he would have been a goner. I think that he was just a little too macho at the time when he wrote out his Living Will. Since that time, a few things changed and he now thinks being alive is very exciting.

Personally, I think life is wonderful and each day is an adventure. From where I am today looking back, lots of things have happened to us. My wife and I have both been lucky enough to retire from our jobs that we held most of our lives. Even though life has been like a roller coaster ride with illness, job lay offs, and all types of family emergencies, I do think that I as a legal immigrant have been able to provide for myself and helped my family achieve the American dream.

A few years ago, we made a bold decision and moved from the wet, cool tempered area of the Pacific Northwest to a much dryer and warmer area, namely Arizona. The weather, geography, plant life and just about everything else is so different here than what we were used to, so each day is like being on vacation. As soon as we found our way around locally, we wanted to have our medical records transferred here.

A few months earlier during one of my routine medical checkups, I was told that I was a borderline diabetic. The doctor dispensed some pills to me and told me that along with a carefully thought out diet, I should have no problem with the illness. I felt great, no problems with my feet or any other organs but my sugar level did not go down very significantly. Then during my next visit, my doctor decided to increase the dosage of my medication. At first there wasn't much change, but when my blood sugar went down to what is considered normal for most people, I started to feel shaky and odd. I told my doctor of the problem and he adjusted the medication accordingly.

Now in a new state and town, we had to find doctors that we both had confidence in. We talked to our neighbors and checked the Internet and found several fine doctors that we trusted and had good relationships with. We got regular checkups from the various doctors but even that wasn't enough of a safeguard so that things would not go bad. During one of my diabetic examinations, my new doctor decided that since my blood sugar was still a little high, I should try these new pills along with the other pills that I was taking and that should do the trick. I told the doctor that I didn't feel good with blood sugar at levels much lower than what it was now, but he insisted.

Walter Willanger

Chapter 22

Then suddenly it happened again. It was a little past 2:00 a.m. I woke up feeling somewhat strange and different. I had never felt that way before. I was not in pain, it was more a feeling of discomfort, somewhat odd, quivering internally, a feeling of dread. I got out of bed, dressed in the dark then walked to my wife's side of the bed, nudged her and told her that I was going to the hospital emergency department to have this strange, unpleasant feeling checked out and then I would be right back. I decided not to turn the light on and started walking down the dark hallway. I took a couple of steps and stumbled, got up and felt my way to the sofa and sat down to rest. As I sat there in the dark, my wife was already out of bed, had turned on her night light and had called 911. She then rushed into the living room where I was sitting and I heard her say, "Help is on the way." The last thing I remember was wanting to tell her, "Call 911 back and cancel the call because I feel so good now."

But by now, it was all over — the discomfort that I had felt earlier had gone away and total blackness took over. Immediately it got very quiet; my heart had stopped. I was dead. My wife never heard a word of what I wanted to say because I was then already in what is known as sudden cardiac arrest. My wife told me later that from that point on everything was like a nightmare for her. The paramedics arrived at our home and rushed in. To have more space around me, my wife and one of the paramedics grabbed the coffee table and pulled it out of the way. Another pulled my lifeless body from the couch to the floor and checked it for a heartbeat, pulse and cleared the airway. Then my wife was taken into another room where my medications were kept; the paramedic wanted to see the name and what dosage I was taking. For the paramedics who were checking for life signs, the diagnosis was not good, all life had stopped. CPR along with the heart defibrillator were then applied immediately. The paramedics continued with CPR and the heart defibrillator time and time again, but as the minutes went by, it became clear that they were not making any progress. A decision was made to bring me to the hospital emergency department nearby as quickly as possible. On the way to the hospital on a gurney in the back of the ambulance, the paramedics were still frantically performing CPR on my body as they had already done continually for more than 25 minutes at our home.

So far there was no response even though they applied every medical procedure available including chest compressions and electrical shocks with the defibrillator. Nothing had worked. So, now they were according to stan-dard procedure, basically on the way to the hospital to have me pronounced dead by a licensed physician. Upon arrival at the hospital emergency department, plans were already in motion. I was wheeled in and initial assessments were made by one of the attendants. Neurological Behavior: None, Pupil Size in mm: none-reat, Cardiac Pulses: None, Motor Response: None, Skin Color: Cyanotic and cool; as well as many more.

Now what? The hospital continued CPR with the same result as the paramedics — zero heartbeat. It had been more than an hour since my heart had stopped and 911 was called. Under normal conditions, CPR is stopped after about 20 to 25 minutes due to possible irreversible neurological and organ damage. All the monitoring equipment that I was hooked up to showed no improvement in my condition.

It was then decided to stop all lifesaving procedures and write me off as DOA. At that time, one of the emergency room nurses who had been in a similar situation before approached the doctor in charge and asked him for permission for her to continue CPR. The doctor gave her permission and she continued. It was a real gamble due to the neurological problems and organ failure that may already have taken place. After a few minutes, to everyone's surprise, the heart monitor changed from straight line to the more familiar look of a weak heartbeat. At this point, 1 hour and 14 minutes had passed since 911 responded to the call and a total of 18 electrical shocks had now been delivered. I was put into a drug-induced coma to slow the body down and possibly keep me from going into shock. A nurse was trying to clean my face, head and upper part of my body which were covered with vomit. The hospital staff did not know exactly what to expect from me since this was something new. No one at this hospital could recall anyone ever seeing a patient survive this long without a heartbeat.

Paramedics' Report to the Hospital

DEPARTMENT EMS INCIDENT REPORT

YEAR	INCIDENT NUMBER	CITY	COMPANY REPORTING	SHIFT	ALARM DATE	UNITS PROVIDING CARE
04	2647750	SUN	E194	C	1001	E194

ADDRESS: 9022 N. 102nd

EMT/CEP: A: 58779 B: 57886

DISP 0203 | PT CONTACT 0209 | LV HOSP 0222 | AT HOSP 0228

EMT/CEP: C: Schaffe D: Wier

SERVICE DELIVERED: ALS ☒ | RECV. HOSPITAL: BM | TRANS UNIT: W-133

NAME: Walter | AGE 71 | SEX M | WT 180 | D.O.B. 6/26/1933

ADDRESS: SAA ☒

PMH: CARDIAC ☒ HBP ☒ RESP ☒ DIABETES ☒ — Cardiac Bypass

Rx'S: Glyburide, Metformin, Atenolol, Lisinopril, Lipitor, Niacin

ALLERGIES: Tylox

TIME	0213	0218	0222	0230
BP	u/o	u/o	u/o	u/o
PULSE / QUALITY	∅	∅	∅	∅
RESP. / EFFORT	agonal	4-12 bpm agonal resp		
SKIN	white	cool/pale →	→	
CAP REFILL	Delayed →	→		
PUPILS	unresponsive →	→		
SpO₂	u/o	94	86	93

CHIEF COMPLAINT: CODE

HPI/MOI: U/A E194 found pt. seated on couch at home. Pt. wife states he awoke and complained of chest pain and collapsed to floor, pt arose and sat on couch. U/A E194 wife was frantic and pt was seated on couch unresponsive.

HEAD/FACE/NECK: EENT clear, pupils unresponsive

CHEST/LUNGS: ~~good~~ resp 6-10 agonal reps. O₂ sat 94%

ABD/PELVIS: distended abdomen, ∅ masses

EKG: V-fib → course V-fib → fine V-fib

UNIT	TIME	TX / PROCEDURE
E194	0211	O₂ 15 L/M NRB
	0219	IV SOLUTION NS GAUGE 18 SITE (R) AC — RATE 30 ml/Hour, TOTAL FLUIDS INFUSED 200
W-133	0222	Alarm room Patch by SW [illegible] BM
	0210	∅ pulse → 200 compression began → V-fib → Shock @ 200J
	0211	IV push 1:10,000 mg EPI → 0212 V-fib shock @ 300J
	0215	IV push 1:10,000 mg EPI → 0216 V-fib shock @ 360J
	0218	IV push 1:10,000 mg EPI → 0218 V-fib shock @ 360J
	0222	V-fib shock @ 360 → 0226 150mg Lidocaine IV push
	0235	V-fib shock @ 360 [illegible]

BLOOD GLUCOSE: TIME 0213 — 74 mg/dl

STATUS AT TRANSFER OF CARE: NO CHANGE ☒

EMT / RN / DR ACCEPTING THE PATIENT: X | TIME 0239

TO PATIENT RECORDS | SEE ATTACHMENT ☐

Walter Willanger

Hospital Emergency Room Assessments

But I Didn't Know I Was Dead!

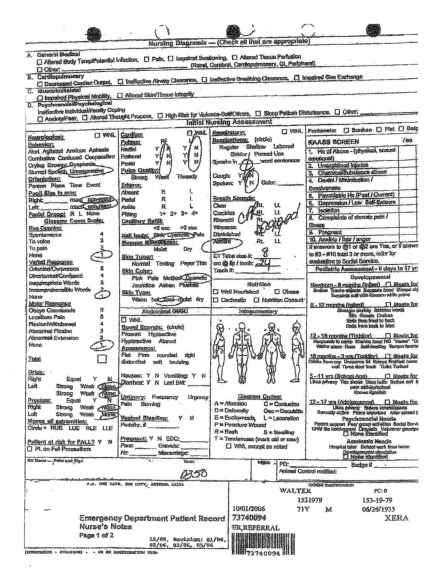

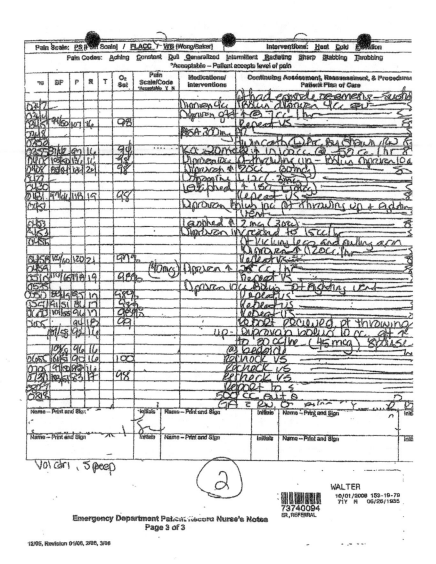

Pain Scale: PS [Pain Scale] / FLACC / WB [Wong/Baker]   Interventions: Heat Cold Elevation

Pain Codes: Aching Constant Dull Generalized Intermittent Radiating Sharp Stabbing Throbbing

*Acceptable – Patient accepts level of pain

Time	BP	P	R	T	O₂ Sat	Pain Scale/Code *Acceptable Y N	Medications/ Interventions	Continuing Assessment, Reassessment, & Procedures / Patient Plan of Care

Name – Print and Sign   Initials   Name – Print and Sign   Initials   Name – Print and Sign   Init

Name – Print and Sign   Initials   Name – Print and Sign   Initials   Name – Print and Sign   Init

Vol cdrl , 5 peep

②

WALTER
10/01/2008 153-19-79
71Y M 06/26/1935
ER, REFERRAL

Emergency Department Patient Record Nurse's Notes
Page 3 of 3

12/05, Revision 01/06, 2/06, 3/06

EDP/RN History & Physical Worksheet – General Adult

Emergency Department record
(Page 2 of 2)

EDP/RN History & Physical Worksheet – General Adult

Date: 9/31/200 Arrival Time: 023° Arrival Mode: Auto ☒Ambo ☐Air Triage Priority: R /Y/ G

To ED by: ☐PT ☐Family ☐Friend ☐Police ☐EMS ☐Other Hx by: ☐PT ☐Family ☐Police ☐EMS ☐Other Rm: Acute or intensive

Orthostatic B/P: Lying ____ P: ____ Sitting ____ P: ____ Standing ____ P: ____
B/P: Rt ____ Lt ____ Resp/min: ____ P: Q T: ____ T O R O2 SAT: ____ ☐Air / ☐ O2 @ ____ ☐ NL ☐ Hypoxic FSBS: ____
Pain Severity: 0 1 2 3 4 5 6 7 8 9 10 (Circle) Acceptable Pain #: ____ Quality: ____ Sharp Dull Pressure Tightness
Symptom Location: ____ Radiation: ____ Timing: ____ Constant Waxes/Wanes Intermittent Food
Associated Symptoms: ____ Diaphoresis SOB Nausea/Vomiting Fevers Cough

Chief Complaint: Found on couch by wife at 0200 – found by EMS
☐ Witnessed ☐ Driver ☐ Passenger ☐ Where Occurred ☐ Eat/Drink, Where Occurred

Symptoms Started: pt in V-Fib Shocked intub'd – unable to intubate
Clinician's space: Time: at Sv@21 – pt arrives pea HA → unk to wife
Unconscious: found PEA on first rhythm 5 min → V-Fib.
→ asystole ↓ LR, Epi × 2, Lidocaine 100 IV → transport police → V-Fib on arrival
of CPR → CT PRN

☐ Reviewed/agree with NSG Notes PCP: ____ ☐LWBS @ ____ ☐ EMS Direction

MED ASTHMA/COPD BACK PAIN CAD DM HBP HA H. STONES PNEUMONIA SEIZURES   DM HBP CA CKD
SUR TAH/OV CHEMO Bypass   CAD CVA K. Stones
GYN APPY CSA CHOLE HYST HERNIA CABG ANGIOPLASTY
TETANUS: Y /YR ____ / N PNEUMO VAC Y /YR ____ / N Y/mth FLU VAC Y / N   Marital Stat: S /M/ Div/Sep W
LMP: ____ Gt ____ Pt ____ Contraception ____ STRESS TEST: ____ /YR ____   ETOH: ____ Counsel/ion Y / N

RN Signature/Title: (Please Print) Tech/Nurse Signature/Title: (Please Print)

WALTER
10/01/2005 183-19-79
71Y M 08/26/1835

EDP/RN History & Physical Worksheet – General Adult

Emergency Department Record
(Page 1 of 2)

But I Didn't Know I Was Dead!

Core Measures

Chest Pain: Rhythm: _V-FIB_ , EKG @ _____ , ASA 325mg @ _____ , NTG @ _____ , Ace Inhibitor @ _____ ,
Beta Blocker @ _____ , IV (x2) @ _____ , Labs Drawn @ _____ , Thrombolytic @ _____ ,

Pneumonia: Blood Culture x2 @ _____ , Initial Pulse Ox _____ ☐ room air ☐ O2 @ _____ l/mm., X-ray @ _____ ,
Antibiotic @ _____ (within 4 hours of patient arrival)

CHF: Hx of smoking ☐ No ☐ Yes → Cigarette Smoking & It's Health Risks handout given ☐ Yes ☐ No

Pain Scale: PS [Pain Scale] / FLACC / WB [Wong-Baker]   Interventions: Heat Cold Elevation

Pain Codes: Aching Constant · Dull Generalized Intermittent Radiating Sharp Stabbing Throbbing
* Acceptable — Patient accepts level of pain

Time	BP	P	R	T	O2 Sat	Pain Scale/Code *Acceptable Y N	Medications/ Interventions	Continuing Assessment, Reassessment, & Procedures Plan of Care
								See Code sheet
					91			
								ECG done
								Amiodarone IV infusing at 33.3
								12 amp glucose IVP
					97			#11 FR Foley inserted
								repeat vitals
								Dopamine ↑ @ 10 mcg 2 cc
								Dilantin ...
					99		intubated	Dopamine ↓ 3 mcg (12 cc) A-line established
								BiChem, PT
					99			Dopamine ↑ 10 mcg (21 cc)
								Lovenox 110 mg SQ

IV Starts

☐ EMS field stick Site: _AC_ Gauge: _18_   ☐ ED stick #1 @ _____ Gauge: _20_ Site: _LW_ Soln: _____ Nurse's Initials: _____ No. Attempts: _____
☐ ED stick #1 @: _____ Gauge: _____ Site: _____ Soln: _____ Nurse's Initials: _____ No. Attempts: _____

Intake & Output

Intake: IVs: _____ cc _____ cc _____ cc Oral: _____ cc _____ cc _____ cc Blood: _____ cc _____ cc _____ cc Other: _____ cc

Output: Void: _____ cc _____ cc _____ cc Foley: _____ cc _____ cc _____ cc Emesis: _____ cc _____ cc _____ cc NG: _____ cc

Stool: _____ cc _____ cc _____ cc Description of Stool: ☐ Soft/formed ☐ Loose/brown ☐ Bright Red ☐ Other: _____

Name — Print and Sign	Initials	Name — Print and Sign	Initials	Name — Print and Sign	Initials

Name — Print and Sign	Initials			

☐ Lives alone and may require assistance
☐ Family expresses concern regarding DC care needs (notify Social Service)
☐ Homeless Lives @ _____

Outcome Evaluation
Discharge/Transfer/Admit Time: _____
Destination/Admit Room #: _____
Report Faxed @: _____

Discharge Checklist ☐ Discharged @ _____ by: _____ (Initials) Nursing Reassessment Completed: ☐ Unchanged ☐ Improved

☐ Discharge Vital Signs: BP _____ / _____ HR _____ RR _____ T _____ O2Sat _____ % on ☐ RA ☐ O2 @ _____ L/min.

☐ Discharge Pain Scale # _____ / #10   ☐ IV Catheter Removed, Intact   ☐ Patient Verbalizes Understanding of Discharge Instructions

☐ Discharge post Narcotic Administration with Responsible Adult & Documentation of Patient Alertness & Orientation:
☐ Awake/Alert/Oriented   ☐ Awake/Drowsy/Oriented   ☐ Other (see notes)

Walter Willanger

Core Measures

Chest Pain: Rhythm: _U-Fib_ , EKG @ _____, ASA 325mg @ _____, NTG @ _____, Ace Inhibitor @ _____
Beta Blocker @ _____, IV (x2) @ _____, Labs Drawn @ _____, Thrombolytic @ _____
Pneumonia: Blood Culture x2 @ _____, initial Pulse Ox _____ ☐ room air ☐ O2 @ _____ l/mm., X-ray @ _____
Antibiotic @ _____ (within 4 hours of patient arrival)
CHF: Hx of smoking ☐ No ☐ Yes → *Cigarette Smoking & It's Health Risks* handout given ☐ Yes ☐ No

Pain Scale: PS [Pain Scale] / FLACC / WB (Wong/Baker) | Interventions: Heat Cold Elevation
Pain Codes: Aching Constant Dull Generalized Intermittent Radiating Sharp Stabbing Throbbing
* Acceptable — Patient accepts level of pain

Time	BP	P	R	T	O₂ Sat	Pain Scale/Code *Acceptable Y N	Medications/ Interventions	Continuing Assessment, Reassessment, & Procedures / Plan of Care
0030								See Code Sheet
	79/60	83	17		91			89 17
0240								BCG done
0248								Amiodorone IV infusing at 33.3
0249	79/60	85	18		98 40	r/bed		12 amp glucose IVP
0250	79/61	83	21		97			#14 FR Foley inserted
0305	91/59	81						alb at intab
0310							Dopamine	albeat intab
0313							Dopamine 80mg	
0323	101	58	93	14	99	intubated	Dopamine	A line established (R) wrist
0350								Bicarr
0340	81/41	91	14		99		Dopamine	Avenox 110 mg 50

☐ EMS field stick Site: _AC_ Gauge: _18_ ☐ ED stick #1 @ _____ Gauge: _20_ Site: _____ Soln: _____ Nurse's Initials: _____ No. Attempts: _____
☐ ED stick #1 @ _____ Gauge: _____ Site: _____ Soln: _____ Nurse's Initials: _____ No. Attempts: _____

IV Starts

Intake & Output
Intake: IVs: _____ cc _____ cc _____ cc Oral: _____ cc _____ cc _____ cc Blood: _____ cc _____ cc _____ cc Other: _____ cc
Output: Void: _____ cc _____ cc _____ cc Foley: _____ cc _____ cc _____ cc Emesis: _____ cc _____ cc _____ cc NG: _____ cc
Stool: _____ cc _____ cc _____ cc Description of Stool: ☐ Soft/formed ☐ Loose/brown ☐ Bright Red ☐ Other: _____

Name — Print and Sign	Initials	Name — Print and Sign	Initials	Name — Print and Sign	Initials
Name — Print and Sign	Initials				

☐ Lives alone and may require assistance
☐ Family expresses concern regarding DC care needs (notify Social Service)
☐ Homeless Lives @ _____

Outcome Evaluation
Discharge/Transfer/Admit Time: _____
Destination/Admit Room #: _____
Report Faxed @: _____

Discharge Checklist ☐ Discharged @ _____, by: _____ (Initials) Nursing Reassessment Completed: ☐ Unchanged ☐ Improved
☐ Discharge Vital Signs: BP _____ / _____, HR _____, RR _____, T _____, O₂Sat _____ % on ☐ RA ☐ O₂ @ _____ L/min.
☐ Discharge Pain Scale # _____ / #10 _____ ☐ IV Catheter Removed, Intact ☐ Patient Verbalizes Understanding of Discharge Instructions
☐ Discharge post Narcotic Administration with Responsible Adult & Documentation of Patient Alertness & Orientation:
☐ Awake/Alert/Oriented ☐ Awake/Drowsy/Oriented ☐ Other (see notes)

92

Chapter 23

The following days were just pure hell for my family. They were warned not to have very high expectations. There was a good chance that I would not be the same person that I was before. I might be paralyzed and in a wheelchair for the rest of my life. I could be mentally challenged, not be able to control my bodily functions or not even be able to express myself. There were so many questions and no answers. They were told that nobody in our medical community had ever experienced this before. Since I had been on life-support for several days, there was also a chance that I might not survive being taken off of it. If that happened, all the problems would take care of themselves. But to take me off life-support ahead of time was something the family would not agree to; it simply was not an option to them.

Then, finally, came the day when the doctors thought it would be a good day to bring me out of the drug-induced coma. With a number of doctors, nurses and my family by my side came the moment that they all dreaded. My hands were still secured to the bed so I would not accidentally pull loose any of the intravenous tubes. Then slowly the nurse would reduce each of the drugs to the point where the conscious mind would take over. With eyes open, without moving my head I quickly glanced across the room. I spotted and recognized my family and some of the people there. How embarrassing; tubes and wires everywhere, and me napping with so many people watching me.

Then I realized that I was not at home. I tried to ask my wife, who was sitting next to me on a chair, "Where am I?" But not a word came out because the ventilator was still in place. I motioned with my hands that were still tied to the bed that I wanted to write. She produced a pen and a piece of paper and laid them next to my hand. Without looking, I scribbled, Where am I?

At that time it was clear to the hospital staff and the family that I had not suffered brain damage. Some of the life-support equipment was then removed and some testing was performed by the doctors to check for physical or neurological damage. Thankfully, none was found. I felt annoyed, guilty and embarrassed just lying there. All my visitors looked so haggard--as if they had been awake for days. For me, it all happened so quickly; four days went by quicker than the blink of the eye. In my confused state of mind, I felt that I had been some place away from my body. I didn't know where, only that wherever it was there was total silence and peace. I had not yet been told that I had died and had been brought back to life.

Chapter 24

Early the following morning as I was lying in bed just thinking, trying to make some sense of why I was here in the hospital, two people walked into my room, a man and a woman that I could not remember having seen before. The male visitor introduced himself as the emergency room doctor who was in charge when I was brought there by the paramedics DOA several days ago. The other person was a very pretty nurse in her early 40s. The doctor leaned over me and whispered softly as he pointed to the nurse. "I would like to introduce you to the person who saved your life." Then the doctor continued by saying that when the paramedics brought me to the emergency room, there were no vital signs.

They had worked on me feverishly for much longer than what is considered standard procedure. They had pronounced me dead several times but the nurse who was now standing next to him just kept on with CPR. I was totally stunned. I could not understand what he was talking about or process what he was saying. Dead? Me, dead? What was he talking about? I was totally confused. I didn't really understand what he meant by dead. Slowly it started to sink into my brain that maybe that's what happened and that was why I was here. I kept looking at the two of them, still very confused. I couldn't really understand what they were talking about but little by little, I started to understand that something serious must have happened to me. I didn't feel death. I didn't feel or know when it happened. I couldn't comprehend that my heart had stopped beating and that was the reason I was here in the hospital. I apologized to them for all the trauma I must have caused and thanked them both for all they had done for me during the time when I was hovering between life and death.

I then asked the nurse, "Against all odds, why did you continue trying to bring me back?" Her answer was, "I believe that I have been blessed with a gift. Several times in my career, I have walked into a room where all the monitors say recovery is imminent but I get a strong feeling that death is nearby. As with you, all indications were that death had taken place, you were gone, but I could feel that life was still near by. I felt we could bring you back. I don't know how, but I had this strong feeling that we could." I was overcome with emotion that she was my lifeline to recovery and I asked her if I could hold her hand as I tearfully thanked them both again and again for all their efforts. Shortly thereafter, our conversation changed to "How are you feeling? How is the family holding up? What's for lunch, etc."

As they were leaving, I thanked them both again for coming and for looking after me. I have many times since that meeting wondered if guardian angels or spirits attach themselves to living people in order to perform miracles. Miracles do happen and in the most unusual places and at the strangest of times by people who do not realize that they have just performed a miracle. Maybe a miracle was performed by a Higher Power using a human body.

I also wondered why among the hundreds of people in this country who had a heart attack or cardiac emergency that night, why did I survive and not them? Why were the efforts of all the other skilled professionals unsuccessful and against all odds the determined intervention of one nurse restored my life? Was I just lucky? Or, was it intervention by a Higher Power? Are we born into a particular master plan to do or to learn something while we are here? For me that night, maybe the master plan that I was born into was not yet complete. Was I traveling over to the other side too soon and it had to be stopped?

Walter Willanger

Chapter 25

The rest of my stay at the hospital was repetitious in some ways and uneventful in other ways. I did understand by now that something major had happened to me, but I still didn't get it. Why was everyone around me on pins and needles? My wife was a nervous wreck, continuously watching me every moment. Why? My wife and family had been on alert night and day and were stressed to the max. During all that time, I was unconscious and totally unaware of the world around me. A little later that day while I was lying staring up at the ceiling contemplating on the past few days, I finally started to understand a little.

Some of my thoughts were "Why don't we get warning signs telling us we are going to die?" The only warning sign we get is that we are not feeling good, we are hurting or in some type of jam or emergency. I was trying to make some sense of it all when my confused thought process was interrupted by one of the nurses speaking to me in passing, "Take care, Walter, you don't want to go through that again." For a second I was thinking how easy it was for me, I can't even imagine what my wife and family went through. Little did I know then that as far as trauma goes, this was just the beginning of it for my wife and me. By the time I was discharged from the hospital, the staff referred to me as "the miracle man," although I knew the credit belonged to the swiftness of my wife in calling 911 and the efforts of the paramedics and emergency room staff.

As I signed my discharge instructions and release papers, I was encouraged to sign up for hospital-monitored cardiac rehab. I was told that if I felt I needed psychiatric help or maybe just counseling, it was all available. To me, this was just nonsense talk; counseling, psychiatric help, for what? In my mind, I just nodded off. Who needs counseling for that? For some reason, the impact of the sudden death experience my body had gone through had not fully registered in my brain yet. It must have been pushed way back. As I was getting dressed, I also noticed a lump below and in front of my left shoulder. "What is that?" I asked the nurse and pointed to the lump. The nurse told me that it was a combination pacemaker-defibrillator and it was surgically implanted while I was in a coma. At first, I was a little annoyed. How could they take such liberty and do such a thing without asking me? Then it was explained to me that it was a safeguard to regulate and restart my heart should I have another episode and that my wife had signed the authorization papers. I still felt somewhat annoyed at having my body mutilated like that. I just hadn't gotten used to the fact that life would never be the same for me again.

Chapter 26

Arriving home the first day was interesting. I felt a little odd since the last thing I remember was sitting on the couch and now I'm walking through the door back into the house that in my confused state of mind I had never left. I walked from one room to the other looking and trying to remember. Upon entering the garden, I was again surprised. I did remember that a few leaves had fallen off the trees in the back and that I had planned to rake the yard, but now the yard was full of leaves. Had all those leaves fallen also in just the blink of the eye? Then my wife said that she had made arrangements with a gardener to come and take care of the leaves.

"You just rest", she said. My thoughts were that I was so very lucky to come back to life and to have quality time again with her and the children. Time is such a valuable commodity. It's the only thing we cannot borrow, steal or manipulate. When we run out of it, it is gone forever.

I asked my wife, "Do you think the paramedics know that I survived?" The last time they saw me was at the door to the hospital's emergency entrance and at that time I was listed as DOA. Due to the privacy law, the answer was no, they did not know. I told my wife and daughter that I would like to meet the paramedics and thank them in person for their fast response time and all the effort they exerted on me that night. Arrangements were made through our local officials so I could meet the paramedics that came to our home that night. The three of us arrived at the fire station along with several trays of treats from our local delicatessen. The paramedics who are our first line of defense had no idea that they were instrumental in saving a life that night. There were pictures taken and questions asked back and forth. We were told that to them it was just a normal 911 emergency call that they responded to.

"We do our best", they said, "but when the patient is delivered to the hospital we have no more information on them." The meeting was very comforting. I felt good that I met them and they felt good that things went so well for me.

Chapter 27

About a month had now passed since I was discharged from the hospital. I followed to the letter the instructions that the doctors gave me along with my discharge papers. I was resting and taking it somewhat easy during the day but at night, it was a different story. I would wake up around 2:00 a.m. each night feeling anxious, as if something was about to happen. I was not aware then that 2:00 a.m. was the time that my heart stopped. I was very anxious and uncomfortable; I would get out of bed, go into the living room to sit down and wait for something to happen. My wife would wake up and follow me asking "What's wrong?"

I could not tell her what was wrong other than I felt anxious and strange. Getting no definite answer from me made her real nervous. After about an hour or two of sitting there waiting for something to occur, the strange, anxious feeling within my body slowly started to go away and we returned to bed. This routine took place every night like clock work. I was now beginning to think that I may have suffered some neurological or psychological damage and that I may have to live with it for the rest of my life. My wife's nerves were at the breaking point. She had gone through the whole death experience as a bystander and now this.

I tried to discuss these nightly episodes with my cardiologist at my next checkup. Maybe he could give us a clear, professional opinion as to what we could do about it. But, we never got a clear answer. We then decided that we would take the problem up with one of the professionals at the hospital where I was taken during the cardiac arrest episode. The hospital staff had all my information on file. Since they never before had a person who had been over on the other side as long as me, they had no definite solution to my problem. Patiently listening to us explaining the ins and outs of the concerns we had, the hospital staff came to the conclusion that the problem was post-traumatic stress syndrome. To take the edge off things and redirect my emotions at night, a few anti-anxiety pills were dispensed.

As I got more confidence and was feeling better, more and more of my long forgotten memory was now resurfacing along with more questions, particularly about life hereafter or life after death. I had totally dismissed and forgotten an odd thing that happened to me about 4 or 5 hours before the sudden death episode. I was sitting alone in the living room watching television when all of a sudden I thought I saw a figure floating into my peripheral view. I could see the outline quite clearly, floating about two feet above the floor close to the wall. It was a lady dressed in a long, green gown. I wanted to take a good look at her but felt that as soon as I moved my eyes towards her she would disappear. I studied her the best I could without actually staring at her. I thought she looked at me very sadly. As I tried to barely move my eyes towards her, she was gone. My first reaction was that I must be losing my mind, or the medication that I'm taking was making me hallucinate. I didn't know. But this was crazy.

Chapter 28

The first time I had heard of people seeing things or maybe hallucinating happened when I was very young. I was listening to a family member explaining to my mother about someone we knew who had died. She explained that this person who was unconscious and had not spoken for months opened his eyes and said, "Oh, how beautiful." and then died.

There were stories of people who were dying opening their eyes and seeing departed loved ones nearby. But, since all these people had died and had not come back, there was no way for us to ask them to explain what they had seen. I have heard stories of people who had departed and would not or could not move on. I was told that they were earthbound. I suppose these tales should be classified as just pure ghost stories that had been passed down from generation to generation, but I still remember some of them.

A story in particular that scared me as a young child was this one. The story took place in a small village way up north. In those days, having a baby out of wedlock was a sin and not looked upon kindly by the elders. Since this young girl who was soon to have a baby was not married, the pregnancy and the birth of the baby were kept secret. The baby was born and it was a healthy baby but there were some complications in the delivery and the baby died shortly thereafter. The baby did not live long enough to be baptized in the community dominant Christian faith. When that became known to the rest of the community, it was decided that the baby should not be buried on the dominant Christian side of the cemetery among other family members. So, the baby was buried among strangers on the other side of the cemetery. For a long time after the funeral, people could hear the sound of a crying baby coming from the cemetery. This continuous crying was very disturbing to the people in the village who by now felt that they had been unfair to this innocent baby. They petitioned the church to have the baby moved or bless the whole cemetery. Blessing the whole cemetery was decided on. When the whole cemetery became holy Christian burial ground, the baby's crying finally stopped. It seems as though everyone I knew at that time in my life had a scary story to tell.

Another story was about a fellow in the village who was not very neighborly. He would always take advantage of people and make their lives miserable. In order for him to be on top of things, they said he made a deal with the devil. The deal was if he could have things his way for the rest of his life, the devil could have his soul after he died. Years went by and things worked out well for the fellow. He became very successful. Then one dark evening as he was on his death bed and a few of his neighbors were caring for him, they heard rattling of chains coming from the roof. The noise turned out to be the devil who was preparing to snare his soul as soon as he died. The caretakers went on the roof to plead with the devil, but there was no way the devil would change his mind and lose a soul that he had waited so long for. The devil told them, "Unless you can find someone holy enough to pray for him, his soul is mine." Among all the holy men in the community, there was only one holy enough and who had the power to stand up to the devil, so he was summoned. The clergyman argued and fought with the devil for quite awhile but eventually won and the devil went away. I considered that story just another pure ghost story, but it scared us children and it also showed us the struggle between good and evil.

Chapter 29

We had a friend of the family who was a good story teller. One evening he decided to tell us a story from his past. He started out by telling us that when he was about 12 or 13 years old, it was the practice where he came from that all the children would get advanced religious training. This training would prepare them for the real world as well as for marriage. The training consisted of meeting with the local priest and reading the Bible, as well as learning Biblical history. There were about nine boys in the class and they all met in the village's only church. The priest was always facing the boys during the meetings so he could keep track of each one and to watch their progress.

One day during the class while he was reading a verse, he glanced up and stopped in mid-sentence. All the color drained from his face as he stared at the back of the church. Some of the boys and also our friend turned around to see what was going on back there. To their surprise, they saw a haze-like figure standing in the back of the church. The figure who was dressed in a white burial gown slowly started to move toward the stairs that led to the organ loft. With the Bible in hand, the priest walked over to the figure and followed him up the stairs and out of sight. When the priest returned a few minutes later, he had a very stern look on his face. He explained to the boys that the spirit in the back of the church told him that the gravedigger who had just dug a new grave had dug too close to his grave. He said that some of his bones had fallen out of his grave but had not yet been put back and reburied. Later that day, the bones and a skull were spotted by a couple of the students here who disrespected them by using the skull as a football. The priest told the pupils that the spirit was very angry and had told him this was a sin and must stop immediately. Class was dismissed for that day and took on a much more serious theme in the future.

We really enjoyed listening to the stories and many of the ghost stories became part of our childhood. As I got a little older, I heard a few stories from my father that I thought were interesting. My father was born in 1901 and he would tell me a few stories from his younger days. This story I'm about to tell was told to me by my father and to the day he died, he swore that it was true.

He said that when he was young, it was a common practice for boys to hire on ships in order to supplement the family income. So, at a very young age, my father hired on a sailing cargo ship that was of square-rigged design. It was on that ship that this story took place. He told me that they had been at sea for many weeks and that it was a moonlit night with very little wind. The ship was somewhere in the Atlantic Ocean several thousand miles from home. My father was at his forward lookout duty station that night. While staring out into the darkness hoping not to see any hazards, he suddenly saw a crouched figure sitting on the bowsprit. He ignored it at first but then after awhile it started to annoy him. He first thought it might be one of the older deckhands trying to scare him since that was a common practice. He then started to walk towards the figure to expose him and to see who it was. It was dark out and he couldn't clearly see the features. As my father approached, the figure just stared at him and without moving a muscle slid silently up the bowsprit always keeping the same distance between them. He tried not to look scared and without taking his eyes off the figure, he walked away. He left his duty station and ran down the deck and into the cabin to see who of the deckhands was missing; but all the deckhands were accounted for. He had only been gone for a few minutes but when he returned to his duty station the crouched figure on the bowsprit had disappeared.

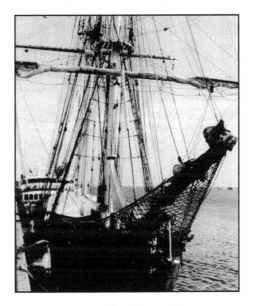

Bowsprit of a Square Rigger

My father noted on paper the time and the date of this incident only to find out later when he returned to port that his beloved brother had died thousands of miles away at the exact time and date that he had written. The last conversation his dying brother had was that he wanted to see my father one more time before he died. Now, was that just another ghost story that he told me or was it astral projection that my father witnessed? Did he really see his brother as he passed from one dimension to the next? I guess that is a question that will never be answered.

Another story I heard was of a young child who had been in a coma for several days. The child had developed a high fever due to an infection he had contracted somewhere. The child was also very malnourished and soon became delirious and non-responsive to whatever medication that was given to him. When the fever eventually broke and the child recovered, he had some amazing stories to tell. He said that several times during the high-fever ordeal, he was flying high above the city, in and out of the clouds. He could see the neighborhood where he lived and people that he knew and recognized. I suppose the story can be downplayed by saying that it was a figment of his imagination or he was so close to death that the neurons in his brain were firing at random and the brain was totally malfunctioning. Seeing lights flashing and strange visions are a process that many people go through when the brain is deprived of oxygen and proper nourishment. Since this was an interesting story, I decided to include it.

As I said before, I'm not a doctor, just a messenger reporting what I have experienced myself and what others have told me. There is supposed to be documented evidence of people who have experienced astral projection, a form of out-of-body experience. For those who are interested in such a phenomena, there is lots of information about astral projection in the library as well as on the Internet.

Chapter 30

Personally, I have never encountered or seen a ghost, unless I count the apparition or vision that I thought I saw out of the corner of my eye of the lady in green just hours before my heart stopped. That is not to say that other people have not seen them. I do find it interesting that the people who have seen ghosts never see ghosts from years ago, such as the Stone or Iron Age. The ghosts that are most often seen in this country are from the Civil War era and some of the early settlers and they never really reveal much about themselves. This may sound a little far out, but until the day the scientists develop a way to tap into their dimension as they did with wireless computers, cell phones and many more electronic, hand-held gadgets that operate on electromagnetic transmission, the only information available from the other side is what the few of us who were lucky enough to come back can provide.

The possibility of tapping into the spirit of dead people would definitely close the book on a lot of mysteries that we all have had to accept throughout history. It would also bring a lot of happiness to many thousands of people who have lost loved ones. One of the most difficult questions I had to ask myself was "When does the departed person's soul leave the body?" Does the soul leave the body when the heart stops? Or a few minutes later when the brain dies? or when the organs start to deteriorate? Where does the soul go when it leaves the body? How about the few who have been dead for so long that the body has already started to deteriorate and they are brought back to life?

Another interesting question is, if a Christian person dies in a Christian nation like the USA, does that person's soul go to heaven? How about if a Buddhist person dies in a Christian nation, then where would that person's soul go? Another thing that I now wonder about is, if we love God and live a good life are we then guaranteed supreme happiness after we die? When do we collect on those promises? With so much technology at hand, the answers to many of those questions may not be too far away. Maybe the soul and energy are one and the same.

While on the subject of energy, an interesting thing happened to me several years ago. On my travel to the South Pacific and Australia, I had purchased a few pieces of native art. I was very proud of some of these items, especially one—a very authentic boomerang. This item was made by one of the natives on an island I had visited. When I got home, I placed the boomerang on the wall above the TV next to my travel pictures. For years, my fiancée and I would sit on the couch enjoying TV, discussing local events or making travel plans. This particular day, the subject of us getting married came up. We had both been married before so it was something we wanted to talk about. One of our former spouses was deceased and the other had initiated the divorce so there should be no problem. We talked about many things that concerned us in our relationship. But, as soon as the word "marriage" was said, the boomerang flew off the wall toward us and landed on the floor halfway between the wall and the couch. To throw the boomerang that far required some energy. Where did all that energy come from? Was there a loved one who was dead and earth-bound who disapproved of the upcoming union? Anyway, it was a startling and frightening experience and it never happened again.

Walter Willanger

Chapter 31

When I mentioned that story to a good friend, he said that he got goose bumps listening to it. He remembered having a similar event happen to him. He proceeded to tell me that years ago he had a very good friend that he spent time with daily. The friend lived with his single mother and a sister. The sister was just a couple years older than the boys and was a somewhat free-spirited girl. The sister enjoyed music, particularly Rap Video. Being free-spirited, she would also stay away from home for weeks at a time. The family was used to not hearing from her but for some reason, this time they decided to make out a missing person report. Within days, there was a knock on the door; it was the police. They had a body that fit the sister's description that needed to be identified. The body was identified and it was the sister. She had been killed by an unidentified man known only as the Interstate 5 killer. The killer was eventually captured and put away.

My friend then proceeded to tell me that the day after her funeral, he and the dead girl's brother were getting ready to watch their favorite TV program, "Head Bangers Ball." The remote control was on the table between them when all of a sudden the channel changed by itself to a Rap Video. The sister would do that all the time just to irritate the boys, but now she was dead. The brother grabbed the remote and changed the channel back to "Head Bangers Ball." A few seconds went by and again the channel went back to Rap Video. This time neither one grabbed the remote channel changer; they just looked at it as it started to slide off the table, landing on the floor a couple of feet away. They both got so scared that they ran out of the room and out into the garden. They picked up a couple of cigarettes on the way to calm their nerves but, as the brother pulled out a match from the folder without striking it, it lit by itself. My friend said that he had enough for one evening as he made his way home. He said that even after all these years, each time he thinks about that story his hair stands up on his neck. Was that supernatural power that they were experiencing? Or was it a neighbor with a remote channel changer that worked on the same frequency as theirs? If it was, then how about the remote control sliding off the table, or the match lighting by itself? None of these things had ever happened to either boy before or since that day.

Chapter 32

While talking to some of my friends and relatives, I was really surprised to learn how many people have had supernatural or unexplainable experiences in their lives. This story was told to me by a young lady who was visiting her dying grandmother several years ago. The grandmother was sleeping and the granddaughter was sitting next to the bed holding and stroking the grandmother's hand and arm. Many of her other kids and some of her other grandchildren were also present, all trying to keep the grandmother comfortable. All of a sudden, the granddaughter was startled, she felt something like electricity flowing up her arm. "Wow, what was that? Did you feel that?" she asked. All the other people who were also touching the grandmother at that time felt the same electric sensation. It was at the exact moment that the grandmother died. What was it they felt? Was it the energy or the soul of the grandmother leaving her body? I don't know.

Several people I talked to have had strange things happen to them. This event happened several years ago and was told to me as follows. The man said as he and his wife were leaving a video rental store, he held the door so his wife could exit in front of him. As she walked through the door, someone else arrived at the door to get in so he held the door for them also. As he held the door and they walked through, he looked to the left to make sure no one else was coming. To his surprise, he was looking at a weak mist about 5 feet tall and 30 to 35 feet away from him. The mist was shimmering as if it was made up of small confetti or snow flakes. He yelled at his wife to look at the mist, but by the time she turned, it had disappeared and there was nothing there. The interesting thing about this episode was that it was at that moment, date and time that his only sibling died without warning. I would not have mentioned that story since I thought it was so bizarre, if it wasn't for the following story I heard from a fellow who is now in his sixties.

He told me that the event took place when he was a young fellow and was living out-of-state. He got word from his family that his mother had suddenly died from a heart attack while outside gardening. When he got to his mother's home, he used her bedroom as home base. He was sleeping, sharing the bed with his mother's dog. After a couple hours of sleep, he woke up because he had to use the toilet. As he opened his eyes, he saw a mist-like silhouette of a woman at the end of the bed. In the mist, there seemed to be thousands of small, shimmering lights and then it was gone. He told me that it didn't frighten him and he had a good feeling about the experience. It was also the only time he saw that or any other vision. As I was talking about these stories to a friend, she told me that she too had experienced a strange thing much like that. It happened to her more than 40 years ago. She had not talked about it or even mentioned it to anyone else before because she didn't want to be ridiculed or laughed at. She continued by telling me that she and her mother were sitting at her father's deathbed comforting him. As they knew the end was near, her mother decided to go upstairs to get his Masonic apron. The daughter was by herself holding his hand comforting him when he died. At the very moment he died, she could see a fine mist rising from his body and slowly disappearing into nothing. "I know that it was his soul leaving his body", she told me. Then she asked me what I thought. "I don't know," I told her. But I knew what she saw was a genuine event to her as well as to the other people who experienced similar events. I suspect it was also life changing to each one of them.

Chapter 33

People have been interested in death and the unknown since the beginning of recorded history. They have sacrificed people, property and things of value to their God, hoping He would grant them entry or let them have a peek into the afterlife. Again, the people who were in charge of the rituals consisted mostly of a high ranking member of the tribe or a priest and the people who were sacrificed were the lower ranking citizens or even prisoners. During the ritual, the person in charge would ingest some type of psychotic, mind-altering smoke or herbs to help or prepare them to access the afterlife.

Even today, many of the tribes from remote and isolated areas are still practicing some type of drug-induced ritual to see into the future or contact their ancestors. But, in our society, people prefer using a medium to guide them. I have talked to people who seek the help of a medium. I don't know if they really believe in it or do it for entertainment. A person I talked to who contacts mediums quite regularly told me that during one of her sessions while they were talking, the medium stopped, paused and then said, "Your deceased grandfather is very upset. I can feel him pacing back and forth because his wife's headstone is askew." This surprised her because she had visited the cemetery just a few days earlier and everything was okay. But, just to check out this information, she made a return visit and to her surprise the headstone was crooked so she had it reset. I was also told another story by someone else. During one of her sessions, the medium stopped and pointed at the lady's friend who was with her and asked him, "Is your father's name John?" The answer was no. "Well, there is someone here and he said he was your father and his name was John."

"That was what my mother called my dad because she didn't like his real name," he replied. I don't know anything about mediums, but some people really get into it. I have had many people tell me that they have gone into an empty house and felt that they were not alone there; they felt the presence of someone else being there. I too have also had some of those feelings. The latest one took place while I was sitting here writing this very manuscript. Facing my computer, I felt the presence of something or someone coming up behind me. On several occasions, the feeling has been so strong that I was sure it was my wife slipping up behind me, watching over my shoulder. To let her know that I was aware of her presence, I asked her, "What do you think of the manuscript so far?" As there was no answer to my question, I turned around and there was no one there; I was totally alone. I mean totally alone in the house. Was it my imagination? I don't know.

The house that we were living in was built in the early 1960s and had a few owners before we bought it. I don't know the complete history of the house or the property but, for the property, all sorts of things could have taken place here during the past thousands of years. So, I wonder, is there still some energy lingering around here from some type of past event, or even a death?

Chapter 34

I have had people telling me that upon arriving at a new, strange place where they know that they have never been before, they have a strong feeling that they have been there before. Could it be that we have been reincarnated and still have memory from a prior life? Some people have had dreams that are so real and powerful that it has been difficult for them to separate the dreams from reality. They would question themselves, wondering if they were contacted through their dreams or visited by some spirit. Those dreams that involve people that we love who have died are particularly difficult to deal with. Not only do we miss them a lot, but it feels so good to have them back in our life again. We don't really know what goes on in our psyche, maybe our dreams are one of the many ways we communicate with people here and from the other side.

As mentioned earlier in this story, even today many societies and cults believe in witchcraft and the supernatural. Centuries ago, anyone who even whispered about the supernatural or witchcraft would be in a lot of trouble. In those days, passing on stories such as talking to the dead and making pacts with the devil would certainly be worthy of some type of punishment or even death. I can only imagine what they would do to an individual such as me, being brought back to life after cardiac arrest. I'm almost certain it would be considered as witchcraft and call for some form of serious consequence. The Western world would have been a very nerve-wracking place to live for anyone with some curiosity about the unknown. That is how it was in our Western culture several hundred years ago. For some of the pioneers who left the Old World to come here to the New World, things were not a lot better. As the population increased and people got more comfortable with the living conditions here, they too had to battle accusations of witchcraft and several of them were put to death because of it. Historically, the people most often accused of witchcraft were young females who were not very educated or for whatever reason were less fortunate than the masses. Those in the community who were looking for witches were most often the religious leaders since they had all the power. They would control people by enforcing strict laws and handing down harsh punishment to anyone whose thinking and processing of information was different than theirs.

I remember reading about an event where some women who were accused of witchcraft were tied up and thrown into a creek full of water. The story was if they floated, they were possessed by the devil and should be killed. If they sank to the bottom and drowned, then they were innocent. That does not make any sense to me. How some of these religious leaders processed information and arrived at these decisions, I don't know. But, I'm sure they were afraid of losing power and used whatever nonsense that was available in order to hold onto it and that included the use of scare tactics. Maybe some of these people were psychopathic killers or had some other type of mental disorder. At that time in history, there were many medical problems that were running rampant and many of these affected peoples' brains. Among these were incurable, sexually transmitted diseases such as syphilis and gonorrhea. One thing is for sure, mental or not, some of these people in power were very self-serving and would safeguard their own interest at all costs.

Another story I read about was of a young girl accused of witchcraft. She was to be put to death unless she could provide the accusers with information that would lead them to other witches in the community. She thought about it for awhile and then she told the accuser that his own wife had also been involved in witchcraft. Not wanting to have his wife arrested and possibly put to death, he became instrumental in stopping witch hunting in that community.

I'm not a doctor and I have no medical training, but I do have an opinion based on what I have seen and experienced. Even in those days, one would think there was collectively enough brain power among the people to figure out that if witches were part of the supernatural, they would be more dangerous dead than alive. I wonder, was it all a charade, just another deadly game to fool the masses and have control? Or maybe, were there really some mental health problems among them which could have been caused by bacteria, parasites or maybe even drugs? Today there are still witch hunts; not of the supernatural kind but rather the political kind. For some reason, there are still people in this world whose only purpose in life it seems is to destroy people who believe differently than they do.

Walter Willanger

Chapter 35

What I experienced was not a near-death experience, it was a <u>death</u> experience (sudden cardiac arrest). I had already been over on the other side for more than 25 minutes when I arrived at the hospital emergency room. I suppose my experience was boring because there was no noticeable change from dark to light or a bright light in the distance. It just got very comfortable and quiet.

For some people, the moment of their death experience is very dramatic. Some years ago, I read an article and some excerpts about people who have had near-death experiences. Almost all had experiences that were very different from mine. Most had out-of-body experiences and they would see themselves in a third person. Some said that they saw themselves floating above their own body, watching people doing CPR on them. Others would be standing next to the people who were doing life support on them. I remember one who said he remembers he was floating and watching them frantically working on him and then he slowly exited out the door and away. Then, in the blink of an eye, he was back in his body again. Then others saw nothing. For them, it was as if someone turned the lights off. Another interesting thing was that some of these people also saw departed relatives floating by, while others saw a bright light getting closer and closer. Although no words were spoken between the images and the people, they said there was some type of communication between them. According to the author, all these stories were related to him by people who were of sound mind.

Since nothing similar happened to me, I have nothing to add to these stories. I have thought and thought about the last few seconds of my life before my heart stopped. I didn't feel my heart stop. The transition from life to death was so very smooth, I cannot say for sure exactly when it happened. I have come to the conclusion that those who are dead don't really know they are dead. I'm not saying that people who are sick or are having an accident and have limbs torn off, burned, drowning and more don't know that they are going to die. To be in a situation like that is an indescribably pain-filled trauma by itself. But, what I'm saying and believe, after going through my own death experience, is that the moment we cross over from life to death is so very smooth that I believe we don't know that we have died and are on the other side. Only after I was brought back to life and was told by several doctors that I had died did I realize that I actually had been dead and had crossed over. I can only compare it to going to sleep. We lie in bed tossing and turning then realize that we have been sleeping for some time, but we don't know exactly how long we have slept or the precise moment we drifted off to sleep.

In my case, when the brain shut off, there was no more activity to record. It was like trying to reboot a computer without electricity. I believe oxygen is the power to our human computer, the brain. There are many theories and explanations of what is the moment of death. Some in the medical profession believe what we commonly call death is when the heart stops pumping, others when the brain shuts down. Without a continuous supply of oxygen to the brain, the brain starts to die and will no longer process information coming from the sensors throughout the body.

Therefore, it is very important to restore a heartbeat or rhythm as quickly as possible. The longer the brain is without oxygen and not functioning, the higher the chances are that the patient will suffer some type of neurological or physical damage. I have talked to some people like myself who have experienced sudden cardiac arrest. We all shared different experiences during the passing phase and also before being brought back to life. But, there is one thing we all have in common to one degree or another and that is the experience of post-traumatic stress.

Chapter 36

That leads me to a story that happened to a couple that we have known for years. The husband, who was a retired firefighter, had made the choice years ago not to be resuscitated when his time came. One day while he and his wife were both on the phone talking to one of their grown kids, somewhere into the conversation the husband excused himself and said he needed to use the toilet. He put the phone extension down, got up from his chair and took a couple of steps and dropped to the floor dead. His wife called 911 and when the paramedics arrived, they immediately started CPR and used a defibrillator in an attempt to get the heart started again. Each time the defibrillator discharged, our friend's body would respond by a bounce off the floor. This was due to the muscular contraction caused by the electricity while it passed through the body and heart.

This whole routine was seen by the wife who was totally beside herself. She remembered that her husband had instructed her that he did not want to be resuscitated. She thought all that they were doing was hurting him while he lay on the floor unresponsive. It was not until I spoke to her many months after this incident that I could convince her that he was on the other side before he even reached the floor. When the paramedics arrived many minutes later and started CPR, he had been on the other side for a long time. In my case, they started CPR within a couple of minutes and I still felt nothing from the first shock to the last of 18 shocks. She was relieved to learn that and thanked me for letting her know. She said, "Now I will be able to sleep again."

Chapter 37

The Sudden Cardiac Arrest Foundation sponsored a luncheon about a year ago for the few of us who are alive. We talked and shared a few problems that we all have and being able to sleep is one of the biggest problems that people have after experiencing or witnessing a near-death or death experience. Being traumatized in such a way can leave emotional scars that could take years to heal, or in some cases may never heal. People who have seen a loved one collapse are not the only ones who are being traumatized. Strangers who witness accidents or an unnatural death are also traumatized to one degree or another.

I think part of the problem is that we are taken by surprise and then we are suddenly involved in an unpredictable event where most of us feel totally helpless. We feel somewhat guilty that we were not prepared for something like this. Also, if there appears to be a life-threatening situation such as an accident with a lot of bleeding, that in itself increases the trauma and makes the situation much more difficult to deal with. I have talked to people who have witnessed terrible car accidents where people were killed. Afterwards, there were reports to be made out and statements to be given. This in itself, going over the accident scene in minute detail over and over again is an emotionally unhealthy situation for people but is something that must be done. Some have been so traumatized by what they saw and heard that they needed many sessions of counseling in order to get their life back in order and function properly. Even years later, something in our daily life could trigger a reaction and cause the emotions to resurface, causing anxiety, insomnia, as well as lack of concentration just to mention a few.

As I said before, to me sleeping was a problem that took place every night for several years. I would wake up and be wide awake exactly at the time or moment that my heart had stopped. I had also been back to the hospital emergency room that had originally received me as DOA. They had also told me that there was nothing physically wrong with me, it was all in the psyche. They told me that I might need psychiatric help along with the anti-anxiety medication. I slowly started to accept that this was a problem that I might have to live with for the rest of my life. It is impossible for me to comprehend the trauma of seeing the one you love, being your husband, wife, child or any other family member, being worked on by the paramedics knowing that he or she might already be dead and might not come back. The conversation that you had with this person will be the last one that you will ever have. That is an incident that is lodged in one's memory or psyche forever. From my point of view, being the patient, it was easy. The actual passage is so quick; you don't see, hear or feel anything. I have many times heard people say, "I wonder if he was in any pain?" Then again, many times people have said, "He or she was dead and never knew what hit them." Or "He or she was dead before they hit the floor." Again, all I can say is that once I exhaled my last natural breath, there was no pain.

Chapter 38

When my wife called 911, the people on the other end of the telephone had no idea what type of a medical emergency she was calling about. Was it really a heart attack, or an accident, domestic violence or attempted murder? Not until the paramedics arrived and checked, could any of it be established. Had I not been resuscitated, I'm sure there would have been an autopsy to establish the cause of death. There would have been questions about whether I was taking any medication. If so, what dosage was I taking? Was I in charge of administering the medication myself? Since we lived together and alone, my wife would have been questioned and would have to go through the whole thing over and over again. She would already have been so traumatized by her loss that all those questions would have been devastating to her. She would undoubtedly also have needed counseling in order to get past the trauma. To seek the help of a superior power is another way that people try to overcome these problems. Others have tried to seek the help from the clergy, but with all the different religions and beliefs and scandals now days, that could be difficult.

Since I have been on the other side longer than just about anyone else in this country and possibly in the world, so far as I know, I do have some insight into how it was for the hour and 14 minutes that I was there. I do have an opinion on life hereafter and for me, it didn't have much to do with playing the harp with angels in heaven.

Chapter 39

My experience was much different than what I was led to believe through my religious training. Was that because I was not dead long enough and I was called back too soon to experience the glory of heaven? It's interesting to think that people who have been killed on purpose through executions are declared dead as soon as the heart has stopped. The same goes for people who have been killed accidentally, as well as cardiac arrest patients who did not respond to CPR.

Although I was in the same predicament, no heartbeat, no pulse, no breathing, etc., and only minutes away from the undertaker, I feel that I should have more answers to those questions than the answers I have. The only ones who have the complete answer to all the questions, I suppose, are the people who were not resuscitated and are still dead; and dead people don't talk. I have asked myself, what is the difference between a living body and a dead body? There must be more than the mechanical motion of a pumping heart.

One thing that I can think of is energy that is present. When the energy is gone, life stops. I have thought it over many times and the best I could come up with for me to understand is that it's like a flame. The flame goes out but there is still some heat left and if we are quick enough to fan the embers, the flame will reappear. But, where did the physical flame go? The answer must be that it is all energy. The energy is switched from one form to another and then back again.

Another question that I have wondered about is, how long do we have to be dead before we find ourselves in the presence of God or the Holy Spirit? I have heard of people who claim to have spoken to God and have had God speak to them. But, I have never heard of anyone who has seen God and who has had a normal conversation with Him or Her. I'm not questioning that people feel that their prayers to God have been answered, but talking, having a conversation with God? I'm not trying to mock anyone either, but sometimes people want something so badly that perhaps their imagination goes astray. I have been questioned by a number of so-called religious experts over and over again.

"What was it like on the other side?" And, "Did you see anything?" and many more similar questions. When I try to explain what I experienced, I feel hostility directed toward me almost immediately. Some have also been cruel and very sarcastic to me and said, "You probably were not really dead anyway." If I was just unconscious or asleep, I should get the award for being the only one in the world who could hold his breath and keep his heart at arrest for more than an hour while some of the best medical doctors and technicians in the world were doing their best to get things going again. But, it didn't happen that way.

Chapter 40

I was a lifeless body when the paramedics brought me to the hospital to continue Cardiac Pulmonary Resuscitation. With the defibrillator, they also continued shocking my heart. I'm so lucky that they didn't stop with the 17th electrical shock because if they had, this story would not have been told. I would have been in a grave in one of the local cemeteries here in my area. So, why is there so much sarcasm and ugliness directed towards the few of us who have survived sudden cardiac arrest?

I do understand that death is a very difficult thing for us to understand; it is totally against anything we have all been made to understand and accept. Death is the final act and that is that! The other thing I can think of is that the hostility comes when certain people hear things that we experienced that are not what their religion has prepared them for. I think that most people in this world have been preprogrammed to believe that certain things are supposed to happen to us when we die.

The only thing that I experienced was that all the energy that was stored in me went away. I was unresponsive to all bodily functions. The paramedics brought me to the hospital emergency room for them to, if possible, restore my life or have me pronounced dead by a licensed physician. Why is it so difficult for some people to understand that? Then, if we are lucky enough to be resuscitated through CPR or by other means or a miracle, the energy that did leave us returns and the conditions to support life are normalized again. Although none of the people who were asking these questions has ever been in a situation such as I have, why do so many of them insist that they have the correct answer and I am wrong? I suppose if they all were factual and correct in their religious philosophy, there wouldn't be so much disagreement among them. I do support the thought that there is a Higher Power or energy involved in our life. Maybe this is what we call God. Miracles happen all the time. As said earlier in the story, maybe the reason I'm here is because there was a Higher Power manipulating the hands and the thought processes of the people who were my caregivers that night. They made good decisions quickly and reversed my exiting this world. Why? I don't know; maybe I hadn't finished what I was to do here yet. What I do know is that everyone involved in my rescue did the right thing at the right time and I'm very glad and grateful for that. But, I did not come back to life totally unscathed physically. The power settings on the defibrillator and the amount of electrical shocks to my system have done some damage to my body. There is swelling in the area where my left mammary glands are located, which is also where one of the defibrillator electrodes was placed. The strain on my heart when the electricity went through it must have been tremendous, but the contractions that the electricity produced are what got my heart going again. There is some damage to my vocal cords due to the ventilator that was placed in my airway for several days to help me breathe. The damage makes it difficult at times to speak. Those problems are a small price to pay for being alive and to have the experience that I have had—the experience of being over on the other side as a dead man and coming back to tell about it.

Some humor has also come out of this episode. A few months ago, my wife and I stopped at a parking lot arts and crafts festival. One of the local fire trucks was there along with a couple of paramedics who were explaining to the public what their jobs consisted of. My wife recognized one of the paramedics and asked me, "Isn't that one of the paramedics who came to the house when you had the emergency?"

"I don't know, I told her, because when he arrived I was already over on the other side." We approached him to get a better look and when we got next to him, my wife tapped him on the shoulder. He turned around and looked at me and almost jumped out of his uniform.

"The last time I saw you was at the emergency entrance, you were DOA. Is that really you?" he asked, smiling. He gave me a big bear hug as he explained to us that only about one or two out of a hundred survive an emergency such as mine. He motioned to his wife and minor daughter who were there to come over so he could introduce them to me. A few pictures were taken of him, his family and me. I thanked him again for all the effort he put out that night. He gave me another good bear hug and told me to take care of myself and said good luck. We parted company. I think he, my wife and I all felt very good about that exchange.

Chapter 41

A little of my philosophy since I have been back from my death experience is that I try much harder now to look at life through what is commonly referred to as "rose-colored glasses." But, sometimes it's difficult and I struggle with it. Recently one of my good friends passed over to the other side due to an auto accident. He was such a great story teller that if he is earthbound, someone will have a good time if he shows up.

I still laugh when I think of the last story he told me before he died. He said that he had heard of this man who had invented some sort of wings that when strapped to his arms would enable him to fly. To prove that his invention could work, he went to the top of a ten-story building, strapped his wings onto his arms and jumped. With his arms frantically flapping up and down, people could hear him yell even as he passed the second floor, "So far so good!" My friend had hundreds of these stories, some even cornier, but always entertaining. I have thought many times about what I would give up if I could have him back again even for just 5 or 10 minutes.

I have talked with people who say they would give up unbelievably precious things in their life to be with or just speak with a loved one who has departed. But, we don't have to give up anything at this moment to be with and speak to a loved one who is still here and alive. All we have to do is take the time to make contact. It's something to think about and it's all available and free.

In conclusion, I would like to remind whoever reads this story not to leave very many things on your "things to do list." I cannot emphasize enough that when the time is right and everything is in order, do it. Hopefully there will be nothing left on the list of things to do or experience at the end. Remember when the Grim Reaper comes, he is quick. He is done in the blink of an eye. For myself, I think some things in life that I would like to change personally are to be more patient, kinder, hold no grudges and not be so judgmental. There should be no need for regrets or bad feelings since we never know when it is our or a loved one's time to depart for eternity. As I said before, the transfer from life to death is so quick that we never know that it has happened unless we are one of the few who are lucky enough to be brought back to life. Be good to people and especially nice to your spouse or partner. If the occasion arises where help is needed, it's nice to be secure in the thought that he or she will be quick to call 911 or another source of help.